"This book will make a welcome addition to the library of any reader eager to make progress in spiritual self-awareness."

Howard Hunter
Chairman, School of Theology
Tufts University

"An elegantly simple, yet sophisticated introduction to the yogic tradition of Kashmir Shaivism. This volume will be an asset to any course on spiritual discipline, meditation, or comparative mysticism."

Carol Zaleskie
Ass't. Prof. of Religion and Biblical Literature
Smith College

"As an American meditation master, [Swami Chetanananda] writes in a straightforward style that dispels much of the mystery associated with esoteric practice . . . . His insights will be helpful not just to tantric yogis, but to people following any spiritual path."

Yoga Journal

"A great handbook for modern spiritual life, both the serious beginner and the advanced student of meditation will find it an indispensable companion for self-fulfillment and growth . . . remarkable book."

Small Press

"An important contribution to living daily life as spiritual practice, especially in these challenging times. *Dynamic Stillness* is practical, profound and inspiring. Everyone can derive value from the insights expressed here."

Michael Toms
Host of *New Dimensions* National Radio Series
Author of *At the Leading Edge*

Dynamic Stillness

Other works by the author from Rudra Press:

Songs from the Center of the Well
The Breath of God
Dynamic Stillness Part One: The Practice of Trika Yoga
Meditation: An Invitation to Inner Growth *(audio tape)*

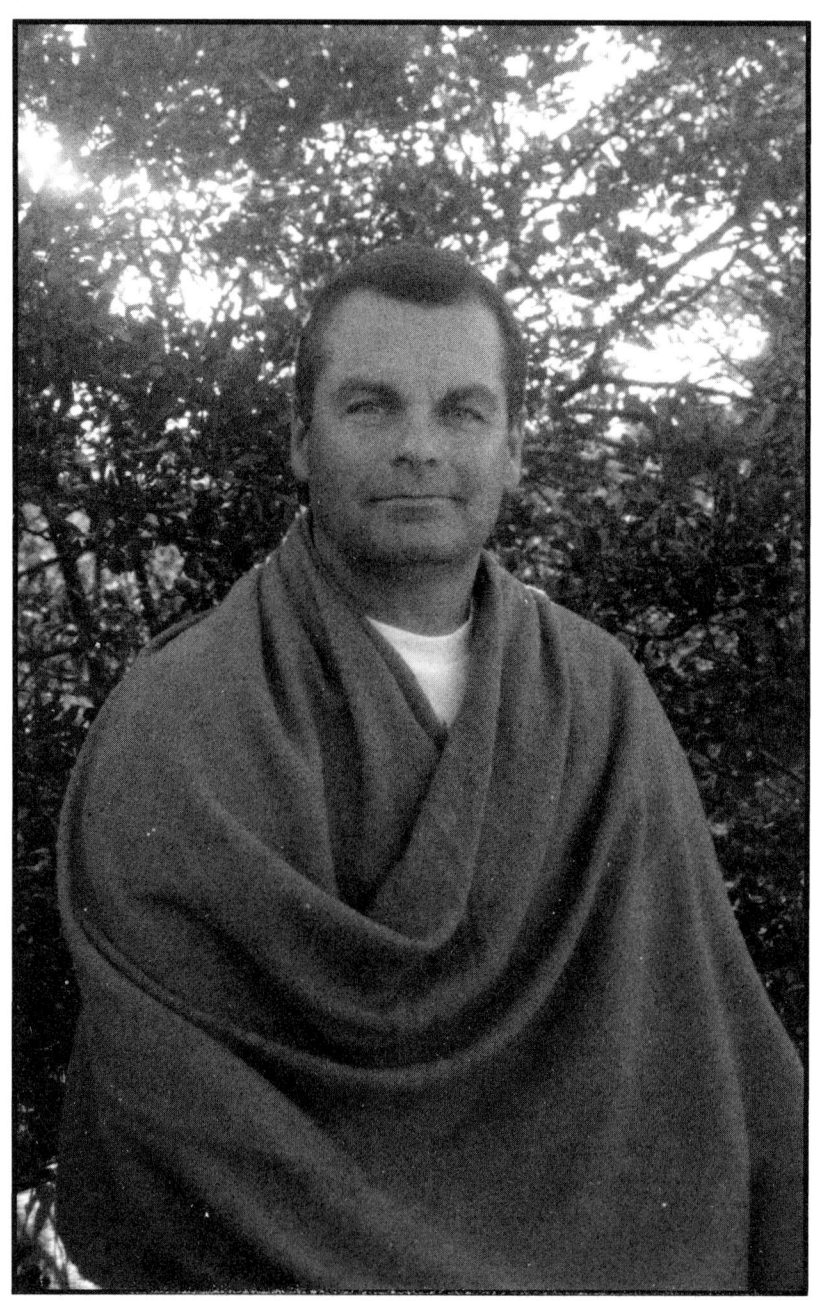

Dynamic Stillness

PART TWO: THE FULFILLMENT OF TRIKA YOGA

SWAMI CHETANANANDA

edited by
Linda L. Barnes

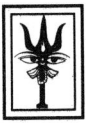

Rudra Press
Cambridge, Massachusetts

Rudra Press
P.O. Box 1973
Cambridge, Massachusetts 02238

Cover and Text Design: Juliana Wright and Caroline Kutil
Cover Photograph: Tony Arruza
Photograph of Author: Theresa Smith

Manufactured in the United States of America

Library of Congress Cataloging-in-Publication Data
(Revised for volume 2)

Chetanananda, Swami.
    Dynamic stillness.

    Includes bibliographical references and indexes.
    Contents: pt. 1. The practice of Trika yoga -- pt. 2. The fulfillment of
Trika yoga.
    1. Kashmir Saivism--United States--Doctrines.   2. Rudrananda, Swami,
1928-1973--Teachings.   3. Spiritual life (Hinduism).   4. Kuṇḍaliní.
I. Title.
BL1281.1542.C44   1990   90-62101
ISBN 0-915801-19-1 (pt. 1)
ISBN 0-915801-27-2 (pbk. : pt. 2)

92 93 94 10 9 8 7 6 5 4 3 2

Grateful acknowledgement for the use of the following:

From *The Bhagavad Gita*, trans. by Winthrop Sargeant. Copyright ©1984 State University of New York Press, Albany. Reprinted by permission.

From *Open Secret: Versions of Rumi*, by John Moyne and Coleman Barks. Copyright ©1984 Threshold Books, RD 4, Box 600, Putney, VT 05346. Used by permission.

From *Nitya Sutras: The Revelations of Nityananda from the Chidakash Gita*, edited by M.U. Hatengdi and Swami Chetanananda. Copyright ©1985 M.U. Hatengdi and Swami Chetanananda. Reprinted by permission.

From *Nityananda: The Divine Presence*, by M.U. Hatengdi. Foreword by Swami Chetanananda. Copyright ©1984 M.U. Hatengdi. Reprinted by permission.

From *Pratyabhijnahrdayam: The Secret of Self-recognition*, trans. by Jaideva Singh. Copyright ©1980 Motilal Banarsidass.

From *Rudi In His Own Words*, Swami Rudrananda, edited by Jennifer Cross. Introduction by Swami Chetanananda. Copyright ©1990 Nityananda Institute. Reprinted by permission.

From *Siva Sutras: The Yoga of Supreme Identity*, trans. by Jaideva Singh. Copyright ©1979 Motilal Banarsidass.

From *Spiritual Cannibalism*, by Swami Rudrananda (Rudi). Third edition. Copyright ©1987 Nityananda Institute. Reprinted by permission.

From *The Triadic Heart of Siva*, by Paul Eduardo Muller-Ortega, by permission of State University of New York Press, Copyright ©1989 State University of New York.

From *Vijnanabhairava or Divine Consciousness*, trans. by Jaideva Singh. Copyright ©1979 Motilal Banarsidass.

Acknowledgments

This book is the result of many people's labors and gifts. For typing the early versions of the manuscript, I thank Diane Asay, Andrew Bonner, Chris Burns, Connie Dyer, Tim Hickey, Jan LaRue, Susan Lennertz, Joel Marver, Robin Mesch, and Patty Slote. For reading and critiquing its various drafts, I thank Joan Ames, Letitia Ames, Amy Blocher, Andrew Bonner, Howard Boster, Jennifer Cross, Kerry Kaplan, Bob Lurie, Doug Moller, Steven Ott, Kimberley Patton, Theresa Smith, and Lynette Ward.

In particular, the creative input of Aurelia Navarro, Nanette Redmond, and Sharon Ward were invaluable in the editing process. I would also like to thank the designers, Juliana Wright and Caroline Kutil, and the graphic production staff at Productivity Press, headed by Gayle Joyce and Kathlin Sweeney. In marketing, I thank Sarah Fahey.

Most special thanks go to Linda Barnes, whose commitment to this project and skill as my editor have made it a fine work.

Together, these people have helped make this book possible, and I am grateful to all of them for their work and support.

Dedication

This book is dedicated to Dr. Rollin E. Becker, whose life work I hold in the highest regard. He has served humanity deeply by demonstrating to thousands the healing potential of "Dynamic Stillness." Thanks, Dr. Becker.

Contents

Preface

Dynamic Stillness, a two-volume series, aims to bring the Indian tradition of Trika Yoga into a Western idiom. The two volumes present a comprehensive overview of the meditation practice taught by Swami Chetanananda, a practice which involves working with a teacher, meditation itself, and extending what we learn through our spiritual practice into every area of our lives. Together, these volumes present what is both an ancient system and a contemporary, living one, with the two elements complementing and illuminating each other.

The first volume, *The Practice of Trika Yoga*, discusses in some depth the questions likely to face a person as he or she begins a spiritual practice. It reviews the elements of Trika Yoga from the perspective of the beginning student. This second volume, *The Fulfillment of Trika Yoga*, briefly reviews the contents of Part One, giving an overview of the beginning phase of practice. It then explores how the groundwork laid in beginning practice unfolds into an increasingly refined awareness.

Part Two is not merely a discussion for advanced students, however. The beginning student will discover that this refined awareness is already a part of his or her daily experience. The issue is one of training ourselves to sustain that awareness regardless of what is going on around us. Therefore both volumes provide useful orientations to a student at any point in his or her inner work. In this sense they function together as a practitioner's manual.

The discussion as a whole also raises broader questions about spiritual practice in general. Issues such as a person's relationship with a spiritual mentor, how one's awareness changes through meditation, and what kind of life one lives as a result of that experience cut across the boundaries of all specific traditions and practices. This book will thus be of use to people engaged in a wide range of spiritual disciplines.

Swami Chetanananda's work represents the effort not only to find meaning in a tradition drawn from a particular cultural setting but also to transpose that meaning into the idiom of another culture. This places him in the company of teachers like Marpa, who brought aspects of Buddhism into Tibet, or Kumarajiva, who helped bring it into China. Chetanananda's work is thus significant to the scholar of world religions, and of new American spiritual traditions in particular.

The focus of these books is on mastery through the practice of meditation. There are many spiritual practices available today, including many approaches to meditation. What, then, have the people who practice Trika Yoga found to be particularly meaningful and important to them about this tradition? As one student pointed out, the underlying question is how long you want the process of refining your awareness to take. The practice of Trika Yoga is a direct approach. It draws on your own immediate experience instead of relying on an external body of knowledge or an external regulatory structure that you have to tolerate as part of some package.

For many, one of the most important dimensions of Trika Yoga is its practicality. It gives a person concrete tools with which to address the challenges in his or her life. The lack of such tools and the understanding of how to use them leaves one with little to alleviate the experience of suffering. As one practitioner who is also a doctor observed, when people live from a sense of resignation or grimness, they do not make the best of any of their circumstances. The highs are too high and the lows too low. What is enormous difficulty in the best of times becomes exponentially more so. Without the perspective of there being something greater, the highs just get you into trouble or mark the loss of the good times as they pass.

Many people are now giving up their successes and their high-powered jobs and are looking instead for a simpler way of life. This may be a good step, but a spiritual practice is more than an issue of lifestyle. The point, as the philosophers of Trika have been explaining since the eighth century, is that spiritual work is not about denying anybody their life, but about asking them to understand its source. This means there is only one thing we can take seriously, and that is our creative energy.

The philosophy of Trika Yoga corroborates this without putting down the life you have to live. It suggests a way to integrate your physical, intellectual and emotional, and spiritual life. There is nothing particularly right or wrong about the physical life, for example, but your practice puts it into perspective. It is not asking us to give up anything but our ignorance and our tension.

The practice of Trika Yoga enables a person to experience everything from powerful feelings of joy to powerful experiences of anguish without being thrown off center by either of them. It gives you a place to return to that is beyond those individual moments so that you don't get lost in them any longer than necessary. This, in fact, is a second aspect that many practitioners talk about. Trika Yoga involves achieving a balance in your life, enabling you to view things in their proper proportion and to rise above the disequilibrium in which we find ourselves.

It is a practice that trains you, instead, to see and accept life as it is. You learn to separate out the romantic, unrealistic conceptions that many of us have grown up with, and become able to live life with less disquiet. As Swamiji has suggested, we find that there is no reason not to be cheerful. We not only have everything that we need; we have so much more than we need.

A third important aspect of this practice is the presence of the teacher. This is an essential ingredient because of the nature of the practice. One student observed that a person's relationship with a teacher has something absolutely real about it. This quality in the relationship is generally something you understand early on, and its meaning deepens as the relationship develops. This makes it important for a teacher to be a living demonstration of what he or she is trying to teach, not saying one thing and doing something different.

For many of his students, Swami Chetanananda is a person who demonstrates the infiniteness of our potential in his own life. Swami Lakshmanjoo, the last living teacher in the lineage of the eleventh century Trika master Abhinavagupta, said to one of Swamiji's students, "Your teacher is a true master. He has the qualities of a saint — he is simple and full of humility." How Swamiji became what he is serves as a demonstration of the power of consciousness to express itself. His life and work make it clear that it doesn't matter what we were, where we come from, or what we do. It is only a question of how open and tuned in we are to the conscious energy of Life, and how deeply we care to know that energy.

The teacher, of course, is one area about which some people have questions and doubts. Yet, as one student pointed out, this is an issue that concerns not so much the role of the teacher as it does the role of the student. It is what you take, what you do on your own. If you are a good student you come in and see what you think of things for yourself. You have nothing to lose, and everything to gain. The point is to try it and see. If you are nervous or skeptical about a teacher, what have you got to lose? You go and check the situation out. If it doesn't suit you, you walk away. If you never try it you will never know.

One difference between this and other practices is that a person is not put through the wringer to see if he or she is qualified before being given any of the teaching. Instead, you are given the whole thing right from the start. If you find this to be too much, you enter into it at the level that is meaningful to you at the moment.

Nor is this a system of personal assessment. With a practice like hatha yoga, you come in with tight hamstrings and are given a way to relieve them. You go home feeling you have a technique to deal with a specific, concrete problem. You take a beginning or an advanced class, and think of yourself in those terms. With meditation, however, it is much more subjective. You cannot tell so easily whether someone is a beginning, intermediate, or advanced student because everything is so much more experiential.

Yet this, as one student observed, raises one of the most important aspects of this practice, which goes beyond mastering a series of techniques or mastering anything external at all. Instead, it takes you inward to discover the source of everything you experience in your life. It provides you both with a logical explanation of that source and the opportunity to experience it personally. It is not about mastering a teaching, but about mastering yourself. Mastering a teaching may be a part of it, but it doesn't stop there. Actually, there seems to be no end to it. Though on the front side it might seem scary that there is no end to the discovery of your potential, this is actually the source of all your freedom.

According to one practitioner, this may be the most demanding practice you will run into, or at least it will be if you really do it. It will demand far more of you than many other systems, because sooner or later you end up dealing with much larger quantities of energy. Yet to practice Trika Yoga in an authentic way affords you a context for understanding what the reality of life actually is so that, given the nature of the world, you can live it in a way that has integrity and quality. You don't tune out in the process but stay present, right where you are. What it comes back to again and again is the notion of quality living, or living an authentic life.

As a practice, Trika Yoga will train you to experience life as a flow of energy, to discern what is constant underneath all the changes in your life. Whereas many practices focus either on the dynamic aspect of life or on its stillness, this tradition is about the unity of the two, and contains all the elements of both. Whatever the moment in your experience, whether it be taking the bus, interacting with your family, or doing anything else at all, you will come to find that all of it is ultimately the highest state of meditation.

The experience of those who practice this tradition is that it is about getting people to have their own lives and become free. What you end up with as a result are strong, independent people. To grow in this way will allow you to feel your heart and to love, something we all have to learn to do on a moment-by-moment basis.

Ultimately, the essence of this practice is that we walk around on the planet with a burden. Whatever the situation, this burden is both real and unreal. We carry a weight, and this is a practice that allows us to drop it.

Linda L. Barnes
Editor

Dynamic Stillness

~~~~~~

Trika Yoga: An Overview
of Inner Work

Everything in the universe is energy or a manifestation of energy, and the purpose of spiritual work is to become one with that flow of higher creative energy coming from God through the cosmos.

— RUDI

Why does anyone turn to a spiritual practice? For most of us it happens because we have looked into many different opportunities for fulfillment and, in some way, have found them wanting. We find ourselves looking for something deeper in life. A person who enters the spiritual search is often quietly looking for the power to satisfy some desire and exercise greater control over his or her own life.

We want the power to use our words and actions to attain success and recognition in the world — to get something out of life. More basically, we experience a lack of creative flow on one level or another in our field of existence. Sensing that our lives are not what they could be, we undertake some sort of spiritual practice, or what my teacher Rudi used to call "spiritual work."

One of the things we discover is that spiritual work involves changing our awareness. The early masters of Trika Yoga — a spiritual tradition that comes to us through the Tantric tradition of Kashmir Shaivism from northern India — understood this. Drawing on practices and discussions passed down to them from centuries before Christ, they developed a system of spiritual work and philosophy aimed at cultivating the most refined states of awareness available to a human being.

"Trika" derives from the same root as "triad," or "triangle," and is a system aimed at changing how we understand the triad of body, mind, and spirit. To say that it is part of the Tantric tradition is a way of describing its overall orientation. In addition to referring to a broad school of practices, "Tantric" suggests that the practitioner is intent upon the realization of a particular experience of freedom, spontaneity, creativity, and well-being in this lifetime.

In the twentieth century, a practice similar to Trika Yoga came to the United States through a number of teachers. One of them was my teacher, Swami Rudrananda, also known as Rudi. Born Albert Rudolph on January 24, 1928, in Brooklyn, New York, Rudi was a person who, from childhood, was aware of his own spiritual potential. He studied with various teachers and groups until his inner search brought him to a meeting in Ganeshpuri, in southwest India, with an extraordinary spiritual teacher, Nityananda.

Nityananda had come to Ganeshpuri after years of wandering. Around him there grew up a community of disciples and devotees, drawn by his extraordinary presence to live and work in his company. Like them, Rudi found this presence to be utterly transforming. He continued to study with Nityananda on various trips to India until the time of Nityananda's death. Later, he was initiated into the Saraswati monastic order by another of Nityananda's disciples, Swami Muktananda. Rudi was one of the first Americans to be recognized as a swami, or master of oneself.

He returned to the United States, where he lived and taught until his own passing in 1973. Various ashrams, or spiritual communities, arose in this country in response to his work as a spiritual teacher. Rudi divided his time between working as an importer of Asian art and as a teacher around the country. I met him in 1971, having gone from Bloomington, Indiana, to New York City to find him. I lived in his house for six months, after which he sent me back to Bloomington to start an ashram and begin teaching. I continued to study with him

In my own work following Rudi's passing, I discovered the texts of the Kashmir Shaivite tradition. I found, in exploring them, that they articulated in a systematic way what I had learned from Rudi and his insights into his own inner work. The issue that most concerned these teachers both ancient and modern — and the issue that concerns us here — is this: What do we most deeply value, and what are we willing to do to realize this in our own lives? Rudi put this question very simply. He talked continuously about our wish, as human beings, to grow. He said that this was our purpose on this earth.

By this he meant something quite specific. It was his conviction that real spirituality is a matter of recognizing the fundamental condition and essence of life. He felt that a spiritual practice should enable us to recognize that fundamental condition and essence within ourselves, so that we come to know what is true and essential about us.

This perspective he shared with the early Trika masters. Like them, he used his own biological, mental, and emotional structures as a laboratory, putting these under conditions of internally generated stress in order to explore the potential of the human system to change itself. He developed ways to keep his inner balance, even as he put his system through a process of total transformation. It was because this process was challenging and because it required a steady discipline that he called it spiritual work.

Rudi said that this work we do is meant to put us in touch with the energy that is the source of all growth. The early Trika masters called this energy *spanda*. They observed that this energy, in both a material and a much more subtle sense, is the ground of all existence. In the individual, it is called *kundalini*.

Their point was that, despite the appearance of many things, reality is actually one thing. This one thing they defined as an energy that is pure consciousness, or awareness. Attempting to describe this ultimate reality, they said that it is both an infinite stillness and a pure and vital dynamic process.

The dynamic aspect — the aspect that expresses itself in the form of all manifest reality — is what they called spanda. They said that this is the essential Self within every individual self. It is the true nature of all things. So spanda is the big picture, the backdrop to any other discussion of Trika Yoga. Their assertion that reality is one thing is what makes Trika Yoga a nondualistic tradition. It is based on the idea that reality is not two, or many, things. Rather, it is one: the energy of what I call Life Itself.

Having explored the nature of spanda themselves and having refined their own awareness of it, the early teachers of Trika Yoga set about elaborating a method for others to enter into this awareness and become established in it. They developed a series of strategies with this aim. In my own work I have drawn on their reflections concerning these strategies, on my training with Rudi, and on my own practice and study of the past twenty years. In this way I have tried to further examine and elaborate on this practice.

The basic method of Trika Yoga involves the process of learning to release tensions within ourselves and to allow our creative energy to flow unobstructed. This method has three parts. The first is our work with a teacher; the second, our private meditation and study; and the third, the process of extending the flow of our creative energy. Each aspect is indispensable in our inner work.

Because this is a process of learning, the Trika masters recognized that our awareness passes through shifts in depth and refinement. This means that each part of our method will mean different things to us at different points in our inner work. Therefore, they also talked about this work as a series of phases. Each phase still involves the teacher, meditation, and extending our creative energy, but in different ways. Each involves a different kind of awareness.

The discussion of these phases brings us to consider what is often referred to as "the path," or "the way" — terms that I find problematic in talking about our spiritual work. While I would say that "way" can be adequate in a loose sense, any discussion of a spiritual path is misleading. It suggests that there is a certainty to the whole business — that it has boundaries and guidelines. If we do A, B, and Zed, we will arrive at the other shore. This is not necessarily so. There is no path, and if there is a way, it is only in an indeterminate and extremely open sense.

The alternative is to talk about a set of strategies, known in Trika Yoga as *upayas*. The approach we take to the phases of our spiritual work is a series of strategies. These operate not as recipes for cause-and-effect outcomes but as ways of orienting our attention in the direction of a subtle phenomenon that exists within us. This subtle power is what shows us what to do next.

So an upaya is not fixed, but flexible. It is a set of dynamic, flowing events in which each strategy flows into another. Even the highest flows back into the first in a total interpenetration.

This approach reflects the recognition that all the elements of our existence are linked as a unity, a whole. It also shows that, in our spiritual work, we are not cutting off any aspect of our experience. Rather we encompass all of it, learning to see and accept it as it is.

The upayas describe several dimensions of experience at the same time. On the one hand, they refer to different types of awareness. On the other, they refer to strategies of practice appropriate for a given phase of awareness. So any given strategy can mean one thing to us at one point in our work, and something very different as our awareness shifts.

Furthermore, each of the upayas has a twofold meaning. One is exoteric, or readily accessible to the public; the other, esoteric, or not publicly disclosed. Traditionally, the esoteric meaning was confidential, shared only with a small group. This was the inner meaning.

The Trika teachers laid out a fourfold process for cultivating our recognition and understanding of the vastness of the energy of Life Itself. The first three of these we can discuss. They are the beginning, intermediate, and advanced phases of practice, also referred to as *anavopaya*, *shaktopaya*, and *shambhavopaya*. The fourth of these, called *anupaya*, is beyond language.

Anavopaya: The Strategy of Individual Effort

The fundamental departure point for everybody's spiritual work is anavopaya. It is the upaya of individual effort, and it pertains to the phase in which our awareness is dominated by our individuated existence. This is the phase of our coming into a spiritual practice and working to attain something in it. It is the process of beginning to work with a teacher, learning the techniques of meditation, and starting to learn what it means to release tension. Anavopaya involves all the actual practices aimed at getting us to look deeply into ourselves. It is the foundation of all our later work, and there is never a day when we do not draw on what we learn as a part of it.

Like all the upayas, anavopaya has a twofold meaning. The exoteric, or public, meaning involves the practice of ritual and any external service we undertake. In this sense it can mean any discipline — like vegetarianism or celibacy, the performance of particular ritual acts at certain times, the journeying on pilgrimages, and so on. Anything like that is part of the exoteric meaning: activities undertaken for a religious purpose. This is also the most inclusive level of spiritual practice, the level in which the greatest number of people can participate and find something meaningful.

The esoteric, or internal, meaning of anavopaya is somewhat different. This is any spiritual practice we undertake to intentionally withdraw our senses and our attention from their entanglement with the world. In other words, it is the process by which we learn to focus our attention on the creative energy present within us at all times. This is not so easy. It takes effort and real determination, along with the cultivation of self-control.

Anavopaya is also the start of the training whereby we cultivate the flow of energy within ourselves and develop our ability to be aware of it at all times. We cultivate and learn to sustain our awareness of this vital foundation of our biological existence, which is called the energy of spanda. We do this even as we carry on with our lives in the world.

This latter point is important. As people living in the world we face a lot of shock and disappointment, as well as the stress, strain, and struggle we naturally accumulate in our everyday lives. We learn, however, to address and deal with these things through the process of releasing tensions and allowing our creative energy to flow.

That we learn to do this in the midst of our daily lives is part of a Tantric approach to life. No ordinary experience is rejected. For Nityananda and Rudi, for example, the world is not something to be avoided, but a reality to be encompassed in the flow of our understanding. This means that we have to be able to support ourselves and function well in our daily reality. So a part of anavopaya involves cultivating the capacity to serve and, in our service, to contribute something real.

In this way we develop a foundation in all the basics of our practice. Together the different aspects of this phase of practice are what is known as the strategy of individual effort. The emphasis throughout is on the work that this requires.

Shaktopaya: The Strategy of the Energy

Shaktopaya means the strategy of the energy, or *shakti*. We could just as well call it the strategy of spanda. Sometimes it is referred to as *jnanopaya*, the strategy of *jnana*, or knowledge. The exoteric meaning of this is a favorite of scholars and academics, who equate this "knowledge" with the study of this tradition by someone who may never have practiced any of it.

The problem with this interpretation is that intellectual knowledge, while a good thing when it accompanies practice, is no substitute for practice. In the absence of the inner experience, any such knowledge is essentially speculation. It must be fragmentary, because it lacks the unity that grows out of cultivating a direct and intimate understanding through direct experience. It is like trying to describe the taste of sugar without ever having tasted it. The understanding can only be profoundly limited because the person does not really *know* what he or she is talking about.

The esoteric meaning of shaktopaya is simple but important. Shaktopaya is the cultivation of our *center*. It means becoming centered in the deepest part of ourselves. In this centeredness, our senses are turned within. Therefore, the beginning of shaktopaya is also the end of anavopaya.

Having made the effort to withdraw our senses, we find our creative energy is turned within, our minds become clear, our hearts open. We are in touch with the subtle spiritual presence of the energy of Life Itself — what the Trika masters called the Self — that is both within and around us. We are in touch with the divine. This is why this phase is referred to as the awareness of the energy.

Shaktopaya implies effort only in the sense of an awareness that we sustain — something like just remembering what is going on. We talk about stabilizing our awareness in this state, which means developing the ability to sustain this quality of awareness regardless of the internal or external pressures at work in our lives. We learn to keep our balance — to remain open and aware of an inner source of well-being — even in the midst of tremendous flux and disequilibrium. We could say that we learn to be happy no matter what.

Shambhavopaya: The Strategy of the Self

The third phase is called shambhavopaya. This is the point where we really discover that there is no path, there never was a path, and there never will be one. There is no work to be done, no purpose directing life, but only a pure consciousness that is vital and dynamic, creating from within itself simply for the joy of it. Shambhavopaya implies no effort at all, not even the thought of effort. It is the spontaneous manifestation of a profoundly simple intuitive awareness.

The exoteric meaning of shambhavopaya refers to the state of meditation. This is both similar to anavopaya and shaktopaya, yet different. On the outside, ritual, study, and meditation go together; on the inside, there is the withdrawal of the senses and contact with the Self. Shambhavopaya, from the esoteric perspective, is the recognition of the infinity of consciousness. We discover the divinity of our own awareness; we see that our own consciousness is not separate, or distinct, from the divine.

In the awareness of shambhavopaya, we become more profoundly aware of the nature of awareness itself. Therefore, we call it the awareness of awareness, or awareness of the Self. We become centered, in full contact with our senses and in full view of all of life's diversity even as we never lose contact with the whole out of which it all emerges.

In this phase we experience life as a great and total integration, called *mahavyapti*. We exist in profound equilibrium, established in the awareness of a dynamic stillness even as we engage fully in our lives. If the focus in anavopaya is on doing, and in shaktopaya on knowing, in shambhavopaya it is on pure awareness.

The fourth phase, *anupaya*, can hardly be called a strategy, because it depends entirely on grace. Of this phase, little can be put into words. It is an awareness of the Self that is so complete that only awareness without distinction remains.

The common thread stringing together all the phases is the intention to turn our awareness inside ourselves. Through the various strategies — anavopaya, which is the same as our material and physical environment; shaktopaya, which is our intellectual and emotional environment; and shambhavopaya, which is pure experience — we seek to turn our attention into ourselves. By continuously contemplating the fundamental creative energy within us, we promote both the flowering of that energy into the recognition of total unity, and our stabilization therein.

As we do our inner work, we cultivate the qualities of devotion, hard work, and honesty in order to become students of the truth and to use properly the various strategies we are given in the form of different techniques and teachings. We do this to have some insight into our true nature — some realization of God and recognition of our true Self.

The Three Phases of Practice

I said earlier that the basic method of releasing tensions and allowing our creative energy to flow freely has three parts: our work with a teacher, our private meditation and study, and the process whereby we learn to extend our creative energy. These are not static experiences, however. In each phase of our practice we will perceive them differently.

From the perspective of anavopaya, for example, we encounter the teacher as another individual from whom we receive instruction. We are particularly aware of the teacher as a personality with whom we interact. From the vantage point of shaktopaya, we experience the teacher as the guru, whom we are primarily aware of as an energy field with its own rhythm. The issue of personality becomes secondary, if it retains any importance at all. In shambhavopaya the teacher is the Self, as is everything.

As for our practice of meditation, in anavopaya we are especially aware of learning and practicing breathing exercises, along with the instruction we receive in chakras and the flow of energy within us. In the beginning we experience these things as an effort as we take them and try to integrate them together into one smooth process.

At this level these activities constitute a calculated activity aimed at getting us to turn our attention inside and pay more attention to what is happening in there. The idea is to facilitate the expansion of an inner pulsation of energy that occurs as we release all the internal stress and strain, shock and self-rejection we have accumulated over the years.

The breathing exercise we do is aimed at releasing these tensions in a way that allows our inner creative energy to expand more powerfully and become a more palpable experience. The work we do with the chakras and inner flow leads us to the awareness of our center. This leads us into the awareness of shaktopaya.

The highest phase of this, shambhavopaya, is our total attunement to, and participation in, the pulsation of the energy, or spanda. This then takes us to anupaya, in which we are permanently established in a state in which we recognize both inner and outer universe to be an extension of one creative force. So in anavopaya we simply observe our breath; in shaktopaya, the vitality of the energy; and in shambhavopaya, a flash of recognition of the unity of all that is.

Ultimately, a real spiritual life must not only have a meditative component; it must also involve our daily lives. We cannot separate these two things. This brings us to the third part of our method: extending our creative energy. In anavopaya we talk about this as service. In an external sense, this involves the things we do for others. In an internal sense, it is the degree to which we release tensions and open ourselves to life as we find it.

In shaktopaya this is talked about as sacrifice. It is the recognition that what we are really doing is dissolving our own boundaries and limitations — casting them into an inner fire — in a process of opening ourselves ever more deeply to the energy of Life Itself. In shambhavopaya we talk about this as total surrender. Immersed in the flow of the creative energy, we pour ourselves forth to further its unfolding in whatever way it requires of us.

Service, sacrifice, and total surrender are all variations on the common theme of surrender, a theme that ran steadily through all of Rudi's life and work. It is the process by which we open our hearts and minds completely, going beyond all our conditioning and all the things we usually think of as constituting our identities. We discover in the process that we are not who or what we thought we were, but something infinitely finer and greater.

This release of what is finite about us — our egos and our limited individuality — is not an abstract concept but a lived-through experience that we both demonstrate and learn about in the context of our everyday lives. In the process, over time, we bring about changes in our awareness that eventually constitute an actual change in state. We alter the internal structure of our systems to the degree that we become open systems free to express the full reach and range of our deepest potential.

This is not an intellectual event, but a life-transforming one. The idea here is that it is not enough to have insights or recognitions that do not transform our lives. Such are not real recognitions. The real change we must make has nothing to do with anything cosmetic or superficial. The real change is within ourselves. Such change breaks the chain of our attachment to, and absorption in, our physical chemistry. Then we view our physical lives in a very different way. It is only when we make this change that we can begin to experience the satisfaction, clarity, and sweetness we all sense as a possibility within ourselves, and which we experience from time to time. We would like to be established in that state.

The point of our spiritual work is to dissolve all boundaries — to recognize the superficiality of all the classifications and constraints in our lives. So we dissolve these barriers in order to experience directly the infinity of our own awareness. The phases through which our method passes are simply the process by which we bring this about.

Total Integration

Often the notion of growing is associated with evolution and stages. We talk about levels all the time in ways that indicate how we perceive the activities in which we engage. This is because we tend to identify with distinct parts of reality and are not especially aware of the larger field within which these things take place. We think in terms of parts and not in terms of the whole. In our spiritual work we discover that there seems to be a contradiction between growing, which implies a process, and the immediate experience of Life Itself in its fullness.

One of the things I admire about the authors in the tradition of Trika Yoga is the elegance of their formulations. Even as they talked in terms of different phases in our practice they understood that these are not really distinct levels of attainment. Instead, each of the upayas completely interpenetrates the other three. This must be so, because otherwise we would not have a fundamental, underlying unity.

Implicit in the three upayas is such a unity. We can say either that shambhavopaya emerges from shaktopaya, which emerges from anavopaya, or that anavopaya naturally emerges from shaktopaya, which naturally emerges from shambhavopaya. Both things are true, as is the fact that the method as a whole is completely consistent with the fundamental dynamics of the system as a whole. There is no break or divergence whatsoever.

There is really no linear progression between these phases. If we are dealing with an infinity, we cannot actually go from step one to step two to step three. Instead, all are present within the same moment, at the same time. Each phase of awareness is perpetually present.

The issue is this: With which phase do we identify at any given moment, and in which will we become established? If there were a real linear progression between them, we could go from one to two to three. The truth, however, is that we are in infinity right this moment. There is nothing to obstruct our recognition of this except the clutter of tensions we accumulate and hold on to for dear life.

This is true of everybody. There is not one person who is any different in this regard. As long as we have bodies, all phases are present in us at one and the same time. It is merely a matter of which one predominates in our awareness. In the beginning, for example, our individual effort predominates.

At some stage we recognize that all the individual effort, struggle, and strain we engage in get us nowhere. Then our focus shifts. It is not that we cease to make an effort but that any effort takes on a quality of effortlessness in the context of a deeper awareness.

There is a total integration from the simplest to the most complex manifestation of Life Itself — from pure awareness to materiality. At each point the laws of structure and process are basically the same. Finally, the highest is always present in the lowest, just as the potential for the lowest is always present in the highest.

So growth is not something that unfolds in a particular sequence that requires us to do first this, then that. Rather all the stages of growth are inherent in us at every single moment. This is why it can be misleading to talk about beginning and advanced students: It can lead us to think that the latter have something the former do not. This is never the case.

At no time is there ever any unconscious dimension to this process. The highest is always present in its entirety. We must understand that in every moment of our practice and in every single one of our experiences, the highest awareness is present within us, if we attend to it. Even if we don't get it — even if our own expression falls short of it — we should be too busy aiming to recognize it to worry about anything else. This is the real way to extend our practice.

What we are trying to do here is something like catching a flash of light. We learn to merge our minds into that flash of light, hold them there, and recognize that we *are* the light itself, which is immortal and infinite. Then we see that what we were after all along is a question of understanding alone.

Beyond All Tradition

Just as the phases of practice are a convenience in the discussion of our inner work, so is any talk of a spiritual tradition. The best people in any field are not limited by a tradition. Nityananda, for example, did not consider himself to be limited by any particular tradition. We cannot exactly call him a Shaivite. We are lucky if we can get away with saying that his body was Indian — but was *he*?

Nityananda was himself. The things he said and the stories about him combine many different currents of thought and practice. He was a wild ascetic whose teachings were totally consistent with Tantric Shaivism. Still, he was not a Kashmiri Shaivite.

When I look for a vehicle to convey our understanding and experience of practice, I find that the writings of the Shaivites from Kashmir and of Tantric Shaivism best embody the teachings of Nityananda and Rudi in a fully expanded and sophisticated way. I turn to these texts, teachings, and ideas to get a fuller sense of what I myself am pursuing. I think they are also useful in orienting our minds and inspiring us toward a deeper appreciation of our own experience.

Nevertheless, I am not a Shaivite and probably neither are you. For that matter, I am not a Hindu, nor am I teaching Hinduism. In the history of the great spiritual traditions, we cannot call the Buddha a Buddhist, and Christ was not a Christian. We don't even know to what degree he thought of himself as a Jew.

We are talking about themes, not schools. This is true even if we refer to the most famous and probably the greatest sage and master of Kashmir Shaivism, Abhinavagupta, who lived during the last half of the tenth century and the first quarter of the eleventh. We are talking about a reality that is present at all times within all human beings, regardless of the means by which they become aware of it.

In my experience, the truth of any great teaching speaks in its own terms. It has such simplicity that our first encounter with it gives us the immediate impression that it is merely common sense. It seems always to have existed. This truth carries with it a feeling of fulfillment that goes beyond time and tradition. It carries the subtle flavor of infinity.

Conclusion

I have talked about the way in which all the phases of awareness are simultaneous and the way they transcend any particular tradition. This is with the intent of putting the following discussion in the context of the big picture. Still, in the course of our practice it can be useful to talk in terms of phases and evolution.

In the first volume, *The Practice of Trika Yoga*, I talked about the issues that tend to dominate the beginning phase of a person's practice. Therefore it is about the experience of anavopaya. In this second volume I will briefly review the major elements of anavopaya. I will go on to look at the shifting of awareness from anavopaya through shaktopaya, and then into shambhavopaya and beyond.

This is not meant only for the more practiced student. Because all phases of awareness are present within us at all times, the beginning student will recognize ways in which his or her experience corresponds to matters discussed with regard to these other stages. I hope the discussion as a whole will not only suggest an overview of the practice of Trika Yoga, but will also serve as a practitioner's manual for anyone doing spiritual work, regardless of where he or she is in the spiritual process.

The inner work that brings about the shifts in our awareness is what I hope to share with you in this book. It is the result of my reflections on my own training and practice and, as an expression of my gratitude to my own teacher, it is an attempt to pass on something of what he gave to me.

Anavopaya

There is no simple way. There is only the consciousness of working, and this takes a tremendous amount of effort.

— RUDI

Introduction

As we have seen, in the practice of Trika Yoga there are three essential parts. The first of these is our work with a teacher — a guide and trainer who is also a living example of the awareness we ourselves are trying to cultivate. The second is our private meditation and study, through which we learn to quiet our minds and release tensions and obstructions. In this process we learn to take our attention into the deepest part of ourselves and hold it steady even as we interact with the world around us. In this way we learn to become and remain centered regardless of what is going on around us.

Third, as we establish ourselves in that internal center, we learn to extend it. This means that we extend our own state of vital stillness and profound well-being into every situation in which we find ourselves. This is service, the process by which we extend the flow of our creative energy. The essence of our work as a whole, however, can be stated more simply: It is to release tensions and allow our creative energy to flow.

The early teachers of Trika Yoga referred to the beginning phase of this work as anavopaya. *Anava* signifies "individual" and *upaya* means "strategy." So anavopaya is the strategy of the individuated self, or of individual effort.

At one time in India, the patronage of different royal families often ensured the material well-being of a person who entered a spiritual community and practice. In return for food, shelter, clothing, and so on, students had to show that they valued and appreciated the teaching and demonstrate their capacity to carry it forward. Traditionally, anavopaya also involved performing various rituals, attending certain ceremonies, and following many disciplinary rules and dietary restrictions.

These practices were aimed at making the student demonstrate a basic worthiness while cultivating the capacity to receive and understand the teachings that would be given at a later date. Anyone who hoped to receive these teachings had to endure long years of hardship and difficulty to prove him- or herself capable and qualified. It was culturally acceptable to put the screws on someone, so a student was essentially reduced to the status of a servant for years before any teaching was given.

In our practice we do this differently. We live in a time and a culture in which it is neither possible nor appropriate to put that much pressure on a person at the same time as he or she develops a commitment to his or her practice. So where does the testing come in? To get people to demonstrate their commitment, one currently popular approach in the religion business is to ask them to pay a lot of money. However, since many people in our culture have that capacity, money really demonstrates very little about how much we care.

In the West today, royalty is out of fashion and, consequently, royal patronage has also gone by the wayside. A person entering a spiritual practice cannot rely on the support of anyone else. At the same time, there has been no other period in history when the value for human life has been more universally recognized and the social stratification less oppressive. Therefore the possibilities on every level for people to grow and attain whatever they hope for is greater than ever before.

At the same time, this greater degree of freedom in our material lives imposes many pressures and responsibilities on us. Thus the anavopaya of the modern age, instead of involving rituals, ceremonies, and ascetic vows, must be the process of developing ourselves responsibly in terms of this freedom, strengthening our skills on a practical level, and cultivating our capacity to sustain our lives materially. This means developing our capacity to work in the world in the spirit of producing quality and excellence. At no point is our spiritual work ever about checking out from the life around us.

Our tenure as beginning students is a purification in the sense that we have to undergo the process of dealing with all these things even as we learn to refine our awareness. We learn to turn our attention inward and stabilize it there even in the context of all that complexity.

This is the phase during which we enter into and develop a relationship with a teacher and learn about the techniques and disciplines of meditation practice. Through our work with our breath, for example, we cultivate and learn to sustain our awareness of the vital foundation of our biological existence. Out of this stage of practice, we become aware of the pulsation of the breath of Life, or spanda, which is the support of that biological existence. This in turn changes our understanding of who and what we are.

In this phase of our practice, we also begin to explore what it means to extend ourselves in service. We start by learning about integrating our practice into our everyday lives. Eventually we learn what it means to make our everyday lives a part of our practice.

As we refine our practice, our understanding of these things will change, but these basic elements will remain the same. We will continue to work with a teacher, we will continue to focus our attention inside and deepen our understanding of the breath, and we will continue to extend ourselves in increasingly more subtle ways.

This is the time when we lay the foundation of our spiritual work. The process of getting our act together in the world; of working hard at our practice; and of reaching deeply within ourselves to bring our hearts, minds, and souls into the present are all a part of our learning to open ourselves to the creative energy of Life Itself. When we can create a simple, pure connection between our hearts and minds, the world, and our everyday lives, then we can draw this energy into ourselves, back into the reality of the highest Self.

The Strategy
of Individual Effort

THE TEACHER

Nobody has the courage to do it alone. Nobody has the energy to do it alone, and certainly, nobody has the intelligence. This is what a teacher is for. And a student is someone who wants to make that commitment, to hold on night and day, and day and night.

— RUDI

The Importance of Finding a Teacher

We live in a culture in which there is a tremendous emphasis on self-reliance and a general orientation toward self-help. We have also seen exposé after exposé on the fallibilities of spiritual teachers and those who follow them. This makes it a challenge to assert the fundamental importance of having a teacher as a part of our spiritual work. Yet I would not only assert this; I would go further and say that except in the rarest of cases, spiritual work of any real depth and duration is not possible without a teacher.

Why is this so? I would put the question a little differently and ask: "How does a person awaken and sustain the deepest creative flow within him- or herself without the support of someone who has experienced the process already?" We would not presume to study any other extraordinarily subtle and sophisticated discipline without the guidance of a mentor. Spiritual work is no different.

Moreover, the process of inner work confronts us with so much intensity at various moments that without a guide most of us would falter, drop away, or even fall apart in the face of it. We require somebody who can not only arouse within us the experience of our deepest awareness but who can also support us as we undergo the internal changes necessary to explore that awareness and establish ourselves within it. Change at this level is not easy; no real change ever is. So it becomes particularly important to train with someone who can serve as a kind of beacon. This is all the more the case on the darker nights of our inner work.

Our contact with a teacher provides us with a living reminder of what we are trying to know from within ourselves. His or her company, more than any verbal teaching, shows us what this awareness feels and sounds like — what it looks like in action. The teacher, by releasing his or her own tensions and recovering them as creative energy, generates a field of awareness into which we enter and by which we are aroused to a deeper understanding of ourselves.

It is not that a teacher gives us something we didn't have before, but rather that he or she facilitates our becoming conscious of something that was there all along. In the process the teacher dissolves all the barriers and boundaries that impede this understanding even as he or she trains us to do this inner work for ourselves. Nor is this something we can think our way through. This is not an intellectual process but a lived-through experience in which we learn to open ourselves ever more deeply to the transforming power of Life Itself.

In some cases we may not even be aware of actually looking for a teacher. We just know there is some kind of help we are trying to find. In other cases there may come a conscious moment when we lay everything down and address the universe at large, saying "I *want* a teacher." However it happens, once we are moved to understand our lives more deeply, we attract a qualified teacher. In other words, when we are ready, we find a teacher who is able.

The process itself can take many forms. For example, I was a boy from a small town in Indiana who had grown up in a conservative Catholic family. Nothing in my background had prepared me for Indian anything, except maybe the Catholic injunction that the primary aim of a human being was to know and love God. Yet by the time I reached my last years of college, I knew that I deeply wanted to grow and that I would need a teacher to do so. So for several months I prayed to find one.

How could I even in my wildest imagination have guessed that this would take me to New York City to find my teacher, Rudi? It so happened that I met someone passing through Bloomington who heard about me and who showed me a picture of Rudi. Somehow I knew I had to go meet him, so I wrote to him and asked if I could visit. He wrote back saying yes, and that I should come in two weeks. I left the next day.

I hitch-hiked to New York and went to Rudi's art store, which was in the Village. I walked in and saw him standing in the back of the store. The minute I set eyes on him, my heart shattered open, as though someone had thrown a rock through a sheet of plate glass, and tears streamed from my eyes. As a child I used to have visions in church of six wise old men. When I became an adolescent I suppressed these things, but as my heart broke open I saw these same wise old men over his head. Within five seconds I knew what I was there for and what I had to do about it.

Rudi put his arms around me in a great big bear hug, sort of rolling me up in his belly as he did so, and said, "I'm glad you're here but you're two weeks late, you schmuck! What took you so long?" Then he took me into the back of the store and made me a cheese sandwich. I asked him if there was anything I could do to help out, he put me to work, and that was how I began studying with him. During all of it, I never doubted for an instant that this was my teacher.

You may not have an experience like this one, nor is it necessary that you do. What *is* necessary is that you have some deep inner sense of having encountered a certain quality of specialness to which you find yourself drawn to return over and over again. I cannot tell you how this will happen, but in some way you will know a real teacher when you see one.

Trying to determine whether someone is a real teacher or not is both difficult and not difficult. In an objective sense, we cannot specify the form a teacher should take as a way of knowing whether or not he or she is real. But from an aesthetic point of view, I think it is possible to have some sense of discrimination. The thing a profound person does have is a kind of elegance to them, an extraordinary quality that we should be able to recognize.

It is like talking about beauty. We cannot describe it easily; it doesn't always come in packages we think of as beautiful in standard ways. Nevertheless, we know it when we see it because there is something about it that reaches out and takes hold of us.

I would say that there are three categories of people you will meet in this, or any, field. There are people who promote themselves as able, who most likely are not. There is a smaller group of people who are, in fact, very able but with whom there will be little opportunity to interact. Still, we can be full of respect for their work, whatever it might be. The smallest group will consist of people who are both able and with whom there is the opportunity to work. We should be particularly grateful for such people and work with them in whatever way we can, because they are our real opportunity. Moreover, such opportunities are rare. To be associated with one or two people who challenge us is a wonderful thing.

When we *do* find someone with whom we feel we can or must work, we will need no ceremonies, no rituals. Although traditionally the teacher initiated a student into a formal discipleship, the true initiation is essentially the union of two spirits. There are a number of ways in which it can take place. Some of them are intentional, some spontaneous. Sometimes it will be intense and sudden; sometimes it will build slowly between us and the other person. However it happens, it is the feeling in our hearts that tells us this is our teacher.

This feeling is the love that holds the teacher and student together — a love that is a resource to all involved and a limitation to none. It is not in any way a binding. Although a certain bond is established, it is a loose and flexible one. It is not something we can take for granted, but neither is it something we ever have to be concerned about finding ourselves pinned underneath. When we really connect to it, we never find ourselves in any way held down, but only lifted up.

Our Work with a Teacher

A great teacher can be said to accept people into his or her company, spending time and interacting with them as an act of compassion. Yet such a person does not say, "I'm doing this for you because I'm so wonderful," or "I'm here to fix your suffering." This is because a real person understands that on the deepest level there is no such thing as suffering. He or she is not here to fix problems that do not exist.

Moreover, a teacher exists to serve many kinds of people, much in the way a fire serves the person who is cold and hungry, as well as the arsonist and the blacksmith. Likewise, the teacher is a kind of fire — a force that serves by warming but that also has a destructive side, with no proclivity of its own toward either possibility. Fire, in serving, simply changes the state of whatever it touches. So does a teacher. Whatever form it takes, the teacher is a dynamic that changes the entire manifestation of our lives and the character of our understanding.

It is all too easy, of course, to look for someone else to play God in our lives. Many people, in looking for a teacher, are seeking not to grow but to take refuge in the teacher's shadow. They start to dress like the teacher, adopt the teacher's speech patterns, and act the way they think the teacher acts. On one level this is the way we all respond to a role model. Beyond a certain point, however, it becomes only one more attempt to escape from our lives. This, in the short run, can sometimes seem very tempting.

A real teacher will refuse to have anything to do with allowing us to escape from our lives into some illusion we project onto him or her. A real teacher will put us to work and leave us no alternative but to face our own lives and do our own work. In fact, this is one of the tests of a real teacher: Such a person will always direct our energy back toward ourselves and not appropriate it for his or her own gain.

For us the point of the experience, ultimately, is to cultivate our capacity for discrimination and also for doing. Beyond that we want to develop a maturity that manifests itself as compassion and love for the whole, even as that compassion and love may demonstrate itself as some spontaneous and gracious extension toward another individual.

This we do by cultivating our capacity to value what we encounter in the teacher. This rests upon our giving of ourselves and not simply expecting the teacher to do all the work. Think of a teacher like Nityananda in the last years of his life, or of someone like Rudi. It is hard to attract such a person's attention or to strike up a relationship. Only when we are coming from a place deep within ourselves and give of ourselves from that depth do we attract a feedback that we can work on and within.

I am reminded of a story Rudi used to tell about the first person he ever worked for in a textile factory after he got out of college. This man had the reputation of being enormously difficult. Yet Rudi paid attention to him and noticed that even though he liked his coffee really hot, no one ever brought it to him that way. So Rudi did, and the man loved him.

The point, again, is one of awareness and not whether or not the employer loved him. Likewise, all the psychology we get into with a teacher — "He loves me, he loves me not" — means nothing. None of it has any relevance to this relationship. All the psychology we drag into it is only a manifestation of our own resistance and egotism. Even when we imagine that the teacher is totally closed to us, it is only a projection of our own condition.

The relationship, if we pursue it, forces us to overturn every assumption we have ever held about the importance of personality. It makes us reach instead for a quality of contact that completely transcends every appearance and every behavioral manifestation. For that matter, once we encounter a real teacher, accepting that teacher in our lives is not exactly the point because he or she is in our lives already. The issue is to what degree we are going to allow that relationship to unfold as we do our own work.

One thing I appreciated about Rudi was that he required all those of us who were his students to focus on our own work. But there is also a level of flow and depth of connectedness that can and does take place between teacher and student that has nothing to do with anybody's individual work at all. At this level every issue of coming and going, giving and receiving, binding or liberating ceases to be meaningful. This is the level in which a genuine love exists.

When I was living in Rudi's house, I was not the smartest, cutest, richest, or most sophisticated person there. In fact, I sometimes felt I was the dumbest, ugliest, poorest one, and certainly the greenest. The one thing I had going for me was that while everyone else was jostling for a position, I was working to create and sustain a flow of love between me and Rudi, knowing that if I did, he would give me feedback of some kind.

It was not easy or fun, and I got shredded on a regular basis. I had every reason for a long time to believe I was unappreciated, and I was definitely misunderstood, because I was a little hillbilly kid, and most of the people there didn't have the first idea of what that meant (although Rudi, on occasion, seemed to).

Still, it taught me that the actual form of the feedback is not important. For example, the Tibetan saint Milarepa worked twelve years for his teacher, Marpa, who basically did nothing but hit him in the head with a baseball bat. For that matter, Nityananda would often curse people out. I used to be literally grateful when Rudi yelled at me. It was better than being ignored. I would tell myself, "There's energy there and an opportunity for change, and I'm being instructed."

This may sound nothing like love as you understand and have experienced it. Nevertheless, that is exactly what it was. I understood that in every instant I was after contact with the creative energy as I met it both in Rudi and within myself. Moreover, the teachers with whom I have been fortunate to be associated have all been endless challenges to that inner creative potential. They have in every instance engaged me in a non-verbal dialogue to promote the unfoldment of that highest creative possibility from within. In every case it was work.

Sometimes, of course, it seems like so much work that we can be tempted to walk away from the whole thing. Indeed at any moment we can come up with ten thousand reasons and issues for walking away from this relationship. Yet with a real teacher, none of these reasons will ultimately have to do with anything. Somehow our work is to find a way to create and sustain the flow between us. This doesn't have to be a big, heavy deal. We simply want to find a flow from which we can practice in a deep way. There don't have to be bells and whistles, and it doesn't have to make the earth move. It just has to work.

One way to establish ourselves in that degree of connection is to be careful about, and devoted to, our work. Only in a well-organized state of refinement within ourselves is it possible to make and sustain that kind of connection. Anything else we get caught up in is, ultimately, only an indication of our misunderstanding.

This is not to say that we will not make mistakes in the process. I have no difficulty with our making mistakes or pursuing some dead ends. Any life full of experiment will lead us down any number of dead ends. But one reason we have a teacher is that he or she may have been down a few more dead ends than we have and can occasionally save us the trip.

The issue here is that we never for an instant stop doing our own work. Instead, we keep our hearts open to every one of our experiences. This is what will keep us connected to what is true even as it transforms every misunderstanding and mistake into something deeper and finer. In the long run the issue is this: It is not the quality of the teacher that makes the difference but the quality of student that we are.

MEDITATION

> *Stabilize the mind in the practice of meditation, concen-*
> *trate the consciousness in the heart-sky; this is liberation.*
>
> — NITYANANDA

A spiritual teacher trains us in the practice of meditation. In the beginning of our practice, meditation is the process by which we learn to quiet our minds and turn our attention inside to explore the essence that underlies and penetrates every one of our experiences. So meditation is not merely a set of techniques we master through practice but the awareness that emerges as these techniques allow us to get out of our own way. It is the inner work that first directs our attention to what is real in all our experience and then allows us to keep our attention focused on that reality so that we come to rec-ognize it in all things. The practice of meditation is what draws us to know the Self that is both our deepest creative potential and the life in all things. Thus meditation is, ulti-mately, an awareness.

But we start with technique. Without first laying this base, we cannot establish anything lasting. The method I give you to practice involves becoming aware of four things: the breath; the chakras, or energy centers; the flow of energy within you; and a sense of what I refer to as Presence. Breath, chakras, flow, Presence. This basic progression is what we start with; it is also what we continually return to. It is as simple as that. Yet when we open ourselves to what we find in the process, the aware-ness that follows is the spirit that tells us everything about our-selves even as it discloses the nature of Life Itself and of God.

---

* Editor's note: As a further aid to your practice, you may wish to refer to *Dynamic Stillness Part One: The Practice of Trika Yoga* and to the audio tape *Meditation: An Invitation to Inner Growth*, both by Swami Chetanananda (Cambridge: Rudra Press, 1989).

Breath

Our basic meditation technique is simple. We first breathe in naturally, drawing our breath down into the abdomen. We feel the breath as it comes to that point, observing it as it reaches its natural fullness and comes to a stop. We relax and pause in that moment, known as a stillpoint. Next, as we exhale, we feel the breath begin to rise from that low point. We follow it upward with our attention as it rises up the spine and passes out of us beyond the top of the head. As it does so, we relax and pause at the end of the exhalation. This is also a stillpoint.

The function of this as a breathing exercise is to get us to start *feeling*. It is amazing how compact and compressed we are, and how little we do feel. When we are tense and exhausted we are a little bit like a bale of cotton, and our capacity to feel is minuscule. We have to take some time to tune within and reestablish ourselves as feeling people with the capacity to establish a finer awareness and extend it. If all we are doing is going through our daily lives and accumulating shock and stress, then we are only complicating our ability to pursue spiritual awareness.

A breathing exercise represents a subtle compression in our physical mechanism. It should bring about an intensification in the energy flow underlying the physical body, which in turn leads to a subtle shift in our resonance, or vibration, and thereby in the condition from which we engage with the world.

As we quiet our breath, we find that our minds become quiet and we become aware of something deeper at work. So the highest function of a breathing exercise is as an act of self-awareness. It gives us the strength to be fully aware in those moments when our doubts, fears, disappointments, and delusions are in play. It enables us to recognize the false state attempting to establish itself, and to deny that state the opportunity to set itself up.

As this happens, we generate a dynamic event capable of change and growth. At a certain point the whole experience becomes nothing but respiration — what I call the breath of God.

Chakras: Centers of Energy

We sometimes talk about becoming aware of our center. This center has many levels of meaning. First of all, it refers to the various chakras, each of which is a subtle but highly energized center of energy in the body. The second level of meaning refers to a pulsation of energy in our cerebrospinal fluid. This is the center of our mechanism as a whole. On an even more subtle level, the term refers to the state of being centered in an unbounded dynamic stillness.

In our practice we become aware of our center at each of these levels, beginning with the chakras. Although these are not exactly physical, we experience their energy in palpable ways. For example, a powerful emotional experience may cause your throat to constrict — you have a lump in your throat. When you are angry, the point two fingers below your navel may tighten into a knot in the pit of your stomach.

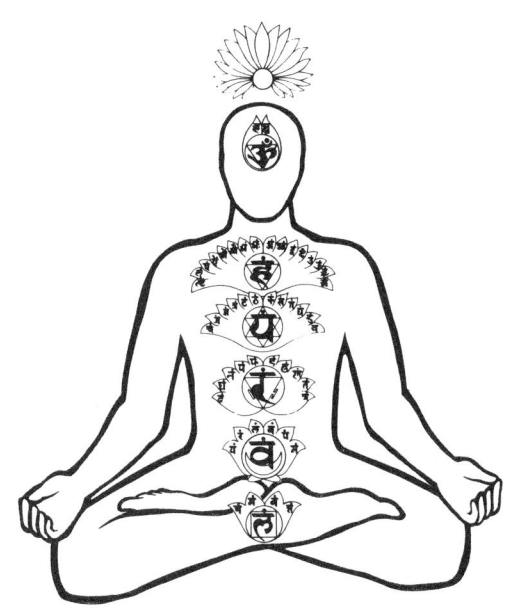

When you experience loss or hurt, you may feel the anguish of a broken heart — the experience of the heart closing — while when your heart is open to someone, you feel joy and a sense of total well-being. It is our experience of the energy of the chakras that determines our state of mind.

There are three primary channels in the subtle body related to the chakras. The first is called the *sushumna* and is located in the spinal cord. On either side of the sushumna are two other primary channels, the *ida* and the *pingala*. These crisscross back and forth, and their points of intersection are the seven major chakras. Although there are many chakras (the texts of Kashmir Shaivism refer to 72,000), in our practice we focus on these seven.

These chakras are located at the base of the spine, at the base of the sex organs, in the abdomen about two fingers below the navel, at heart level in the center of the chest, in the throat, between the eyes, and at the top of the head.

Trika Yoga is the practice by which we cultivate our awareness of these chakras and of the energy flow within and between them. When we sit in meditation, we bring our attention to these centers, and our very attention causes them to open. This means that we experience the chakras most strongly whenever we find that place within ourselves where we experience a certain level of relaxation, openness, and sweetness.

Only when we get caught up in our tensions do we begin to close ourselves off in various ways that obstruct this awareness. These tensions disturb our capacity to open ourselves to our lives as they are, and to explore our true potential. Instead of being able to observe the depth to which we can open, we surround ourselves with blockades and barriers. We reject everything and shut down. So the issue in every aspect of our work with the chakras is one of openness.

Flow: Experiencing the Circulation of the Energy

While each of the chakras is important in the process of refining our awareness, even more important is the flow of energy between them to which we become sensitive. This flow is actually a circuit that goes down the front of our body through the chakras and then rises up the spinal column through the top of the head. We do not create this circuit; it already exists. We simply work to cultivate our awareness of it.

As we do this we gradually withdraw the focus of our attention from the physical world and take it within ourselves. Even as we interact with the world, we become more and more attuned to the energy that is its support. We become aware of two dimensions of our experience at the same time. In this way the chakras are the gateways between our inner and outer experiences.

Breath is the vehicle by which we experience this flow within and between the chakras. First we learn to focus our attention on the breath; then we expand our awareness to include the chakras. We learn to follow the flow between them and feel the energy pierce the centers of the chakras, rise up the spinal column to the top of the head, only to flow down again in an unbroken process. This is the energy called kundalini, the expression of the pulsation of Life Itself on an individualized level.

The experience of this flow can be a quiet one, and you may not feel it for a while. If you have never paid attention to your breath, the chakras, or the experience of flow, it takes time to reorient your attention to notice what are fundamentally subtle events. So your effort is to become quiet enough to notice them. At the same time, whether you are conscious of being aware of them or not, they are always happening. As you do become aware, even that awareness will undergo many refinements over time.

The experience of this flow in all its dimensions changes us deeply. For example, it dissolves what we ordinarily think of as knowledge. It does so by deepening our understanding and, in the process, putting an end to what we think of as knowable. As we become increasingly aware of the underlying unity of all experience, we are less and less concerned with the apparent distinctions and separations between things as subjects and objects.

This is something we cannot grasp intellectually. Even better than talking about it is simply doing it over and over again, until you have refined your understanding to the point that the true grain of it comes clear to you. This is because self-awareness goes to self-awareness. When we are in a state of real openness, everything finds its balance and vibrates according to its own nature in proper relationship to every other pattern around it. Then we are not polluting our environment with our desires and misunderstanding. We see things as they are, and not as we want them to be.

Eventually we realize that if there is only one thing, then from the perspective of the highest reality there is no such thing as flow from one point to another. Nevertheless, we talk about flow to put ourselves in touch with the deeper reality that we are. But the real flow is the flow of our attention. Like the beam of a spotlight, we focus first here, then there. Ultimately, we forget about flow and find within it the experience of harmony and stillness in the unity of the Self.

Presence

When we become still, we begin to notice a kind of presence. I use the term "Presence" because we can actually sense it. If we pay attention to it, we discover that there are many levels of fluctuation within it. Moreover, as we stabilize our individual awareness within that field, something about it opens up in every direction. This experience of Presence is known as *samadhi*.

As our hearts open and we begin to experience the joy implicit within the flow, our awareness of our connection to the whole intensifies. We learn to sustain this perception even as we observe various differentiated events operating within the field of our awareness. Having awakened our creative energy and cultivated its flow, we recognize our bodies, minds, and every other aspect of ourselves to be nothing but creative energy. Eventually we discover the same to be true of every other body and we see our fundamental unity in Life Itself.

We come to understand that we are really everything that is. There is nothing we have to change, nothing we have to do. There is no place to go. There is only this knowing of the Self. Experiencing the Self as it is, infinite and without boundaries, we feel a sense of fullness and ease, quiet and total well-being. This is the direct experience of the Self, which we call Presence.

This is not a denial of the body but a celebration of it. It is not a denial of the mind, but the joy within the mind. It is not the end of breathing but the very power within the breath. A person established in the Presence understands the whole world to be a celebration, an expression of the love of God.

The Importance of Practice

Think about what distinguishes a person going to his or her first violin lesson from a universally recognized master of the violin. I would suggest that one difference lies in the extent and nature of their practice. The effort that a beginning person makes on the first day and the effort of the greatest master on earth are exactly the same. The difference is that the beginning student has not yet trained all his or her reflexes and responses. A master, on the other hand, has all of those skills and, in addition, can coax from the instrument tones that it was not even designed to produce. Likewise, we have within us possibilities not imagined by most people.

Practice is literally a matter of putting our fingers on the strings, feeling the vibration, listening to the tones, feeling again and again, and hearing from every direction. The master does not cease to finger the strings or move the bow. In fact, this is always the foundation of what he or she does with an increasing depth of skill.

So whether we are talking about the first day or the last, it is the depth of the time we spend and the quality of the understanding we develop through practice that translate into the potential for transformation in the field of our lives. This makes practice totally important. It is, and remains, the essence of our inner work. If we are ever to understand the subtlety and power of surrender — an idea to which we will return over and over again in the discussion that follows — we must practice.

This may not necessarily mean that we spend two hours a day in meditation, or that we sit twice a day. It is a good thing to practice at least once daily, but sometimes even that may not be possible. In one sense, sitting is not even the essence of practice. Rather it is our awareness and experience of flow working themselves ever deeper.

This whole process should mature us. Instead of making us closed or cynical toward life, it should make us professionals in our work and seasoned in the context of our practice. So in a sense I am giving you a justification for maintaining your commitment to practicing at all times, persevering through every difficulty, and keeping your heart and mind open as you work to sustain the flow every day.

The issue of continuing to practice is also a subtle one because, in spiritual work, people sometimes imagine they are practicing when they actually are not. It can happen, for example, when a person has strong results from a particular technique. This is why a little bit of success with a technique can be a tricky thing. Our tendency will be to stay with the technique and be limited by it, inadvertently creating a resistance to many other, different levels of appreciation.

It is easy to become comfortable where we are and not push ourselves to new levels of experience. We can notice this in terms of the things to which we have a lot of resistance. This makes our resistance often a good indication of where we need to change our approach.

I observe that people who have accomplished something often stop learning from it and depend, instead, on doing the same thing over and over again. This may be something that worked and was useful ten years before, but that is now really out of touch with the process. That is, their awareness has become so sloppy that their work has nothing to do with the situation to which they are now relating.

Unfortunately, we are conditioned by most of our experience to think that we can work and then relax. So we tend to work very hard and then blow everything off whenever we can. We don't allow ourselves to become established in a deeper awareness and we don't bring our training to work in the whole field of our lives.

For that matter, it doesn't take all that long to fall out of touch. It is like me with basketball: I go out to the court thinking it has only been a couple of years since I last played (when "only a couple of years" is actually something like twelve). But, no problem — I can get out there and do it! So I start dribbling around and making one of those old moves I used to make with great speed and ease, moving toward the shot I used to hit every time. First of all, however, I end up kicking the ball. The second time, I walk through the lay-up at about ten percent of the appropriate speed, and when I *do* take the shot, I miss the backboard. There is no substitute for practice.

A lot of time and effort go into our inner work. There is little possibility that a person who hasn't practiced will be able to sustain a deeper condition of recognition over time. Think of all those occasions in your life when you have had some kind of powerful insight and said to yourself, "I must remember this forever." Two days later it is gone.

The transformation of information from the short-term to the long-term memory is based on a chemical change in the nervous system. From the point of view of spiritual growth, the chemical change is so fine that by the time our minds figure it out it will probably have been there for five years. It is not a question of conceptual or ideational information. It is simply awareness. This is a subtlety that transcends the mind. So if you are trying to use the mind to figure it out, you are basically wading around in the barnyard.

There is neither psychological content nor mental knowledge to what you will learn in your spiritual work. The lessons are implicit in the chemical change. Indeed, true learning is based on deep chemical change. Some of the things you learn you will never be able to articulate because there are no words with which to do so. When you sit in meditation, you absorb and internalize these experiences, making them your own without their ever even touching your mind in the slightest.

For that matter, much of what we articulate at this level is nonverbal. It is the most powerful and important form of articulation. It involves being centered within ourselves and open to whoever is around us. This is not simply a matter of joining them but of sharing, even as we remain strong within our own center. This requires training.

If we are going to absorb these transpersonal energies and universal forces into our biological mechanisms in such a way that our bodies and brains can be informed of them and support our further evolvement, it will take time. It takes time for our bodies and brain cells to become attuned to those higher frequencies. The peeling away of shocks and strains requires real circumstances and a real understanding on our part.

When Rudi spoke about planting a seed in someone that would only manifest after fifteen years, he was expressing something that was absolutely true. It is only if we continue to work for years that we get a real handle on the things that were transmitted to us ten years ago. If we quit working, we lose information we never knew we had in the first place.

It is difficult to overestimate the number of hours of quiet inner work it takes to acquire confidence, strength, and stability in the experience and awareness of our deepest creative energy. It takes many hours and a lot of work. This doesn't necessarily mean that we actually have to sit for all those hours; it does mean we have to find a way to be quiet, go inside, and sit with the deepest inner resonance we can connect to.

As we do so, we have to maintain our awareness of that resonance. This is really the essence of changing our chemistry. It is in this chemical change that we come to the possibility of shedding our attachments and transforming our lives.

By sitting quietly in that experience, we find that slowly it unwinds and reveals itself. It comes to us and exposes its infinite nature. By going into that state over and over again, we allow every part of us — our bodies, brains, and cells — to be educated to the existence of the inner Self. Like plants under the sun, we bend toward the experience of that inner light.

Real potential takes a long time to develop and can take some pretty circuitous routes as it unfolds. So we cannot think in terms of straight lines, or of cause and effect. Here there are no straight lines going anywhere. In fact, people who try to push anything along a straight line push everything over the cliff.

Running through the events and circumstances of our lives is a mystical reality that we are attempting to unfold. It has nothing to do with events or circumstances and everything to do with shedding our illusions and delusions. It involves changing our chemistry to the extent that it can sustain increasingly higher and finer energies.

As we master the techniques of our method and begin to use them in the context of the different situations of our daily lives, we begin to experience a process unfolding within us, transforming the patterns of our lives. This brings us into contact with our essential state and the recognition that it is unbounded in any way.

This transcendence of our boundaries is a joyous occasion. Abhinavagupta says that it is not like drinking wine or making love. It is not like the ecstasy that is sometimes promoted as the object of spiritual attainment or that is sometimes even a part of spiritual experience. Rather, he says, this is a joy comparable to the release of a burden. This peace allows for the stable and enduring experience of our unlimited essence. In that state we are completely free.

EXTENDING THE ENERGY: SERVICE

*Always taste peace and abstain from useless chatter. Avoid
the expressions "Who are you, why, how, what is that?"
They clutter the path. What is then revealed is the light
which illuminates the distinction between existence and
nonexistence. It is the way without division, the domain
of Shiva.*

— ABHINAVAGUPTA

Releasing Tensions . . .

The challenge we face every day is to learn to stay open
and probe the depth of our potential, to learn to release our
tensions and allow our creative energy to flow. This is a simple idea, but it is the very crux of our well-being. What limits
us in unfolding the potential of our mechanism is the continuous stress and strain we sustain as human beings. We can also
call it conditioning: We are conditioned to function in certain
ways. We do so, and the world rewards us for certain forms of
behavior.

What no one ever tells us is that whenever we plug into
the world we put stress on our systems. The minute we identify with anything — any concept, idea, or perception — we
are taking in pure energy and giving it some structure. In this
way we gradually construct a whole series of compensatory
mechanisms. What we rarely see is that it is really our own
misunderstandings that we are projecting onto some situation.

Any tension we experience represents the measure of our
ability to recognize, release, and express the creative energy of
Life Itself. On the one hand, we confront internal tensions in
our fears, doubts, and insecurities, all of which derive from the
concepts we hold about reality. On the other hand, we also
face external tensions in the unfulfilled expectations of others.

How do these different tensions function? Our inner tensions cause us to view things from a skewed perspective and
react inappropriately to the buildup of the energy within us.
We draw faulty distinctions, as in the example frequently used

in Indian philosophy of someone's mistaking a rope for a serpent and reacting to it as though it were the latter. Our external tensions are the pressures exerted on us by our environment — what we could call the different atmospheric pressures in our lives. An external tension for us is often the result of a tension that is internal for someone else.

The main thing, though, is that any tension, regardless of the details, is crystallized energy. In every case it has a certain magnetism to it. That is, it attracts one thing and repels another. These attractions and aversions are the source of our thoughts, emotions, and actions. As long as we carry a sense of attraction and aversion, we see the world in terms of our desires and fears, our wants and needs. We don't understand that both sides of the coin are nothing more than our tensions extended through our sensory apprehensions of the world.

Nor do we realize that we have a choice in how to respond to the situations we encounter. In any tense situation, everybody usually dives for the lowest level of operation. Rarely do we see people trying to be loving or looking to understand the interests that will best serve the whole event. To do that requires not only that we be centered but that we keep our hearts open at the same time. Then we know who we are and what our work is. We can be strong in that awareness and at the same time discern the needs of the whole and try to promote that whole.

In a larger sense, any difficult situation gives us the opportunity to choose what our lives will be. It is all too easy to be magnetized by the lowest level available in a situation. Most of us are constantly seeking a common denominator as a basis for interaction. But if we only cultivate what is common, we will be trapped in a common life and never discover a life that is extraordinary.

In fact, people often get so crystallized in their tensions that they end up living lives in which they merely endure difficulty, unaware of the extent to which they have choices in the matter. Part of the problem with simply enduring difficulty, however, is that a psychological mechanism gets established within us that begins a steady broadcast to ourselves and others. It says, "I can't really deal with this." Such a message both feeds on, and reinforces, itself. It relegates us to the realm of incompetence and denies our true capability. Whenever we get caught up in such mental and emotional complexity we are consumed by it, because tensions of this kind are voracious. They eat everything, especially us.

We have to recognize that once we kick a particular dynamic into motion it sets a corresponding psychology in motion. In other words, after we fire the gun there is little we can do except hope that our aim was true — or not true, depending on what we decide after we pull the trigger.

As we come to recognize everything to be an extension of ourselves, we see that the various tensions and judgments we experience are our own issue. Then it is up to us to dissolve them in a simple way. The basic question is whether something is a part of our lives or not. Is it worth doing, or not? If it is, then there is no need to talk about it. We just do it. If it is not, then what are we going on about?

Any time we bump into a struggle of any kind, we have to pull back and ask what we are really struggling with. For the most part the struggle is never about what we think it is. We fight about things that are, essentially, not up to us because we don't have the strength to engage in the real issue. So there is a two-part process involved in going beyond this dynamic: First, we stop fighting; second, we allow the real question to engage within us.

Generally speaking there is a ten-to-one ratio between the events we should ignore and those to which we should respond. In fact, many of the disturbances we experience we *can* ignore. There are only a few we cannot. It helps to remember that each situation that presents itself in our lives is a blessing that could nourish us deeply and also complete certain patterns in us so that we are free to continue growing. We can make any event either a support to the process of growing or a circuit breaker by which strong energies are interrupted and dissipated. This is up to us.

I, myself, was trained to do what Rudi used to call "eating tensions" when confronting strong situations. By this he meant connecting to them and absorbing them without ever losing awareness of an ultimate unity. So we become almost professional about opening to strong energies and absorbing them, remaining centered even while they do their tap dance on our nerves to reorganize us. The more we learn to release tensions and allow our creative energy to flow freely, the more we discover the importance of absorbing every strong energy into ourselves.

As this happens we find that everything we *do* is actually a process of working with energy. This is unavoidable. When we understand this we bring a different level of awareness to every activity we undertake. We release the crystallization in which we get involved when we are locked into our more superficial perception of events in the world. We want to look more deeply than that. No matter what work we are doing, we want to be increasingly concerned with its energy so that we can operate with a deeper insight, oriented by a deeper perspective.

If we are going to have this experience and sustain it, we cannot be reacting to everything that is going on around us. We cannot be wondering what this one thinks of us or what that one thinks. We have to rise above all the "why this, and why that?" Otherwise, we only get lost in screwing our own heads around. When the field of energy around us contracts, our work is to be on the alert and release that contraction over and over again, so that we can spin *it* around.

When someone does something that disturbs us, our own disturbance is really only a matter of some tension within us resonating with that tension. Perhaps the tension in us even precedes the actual disturbance. Because it is present in us already, we view the situations around us through these tension glasses and see them in ways that have nothing to do with how they really are.

All we are then doing is building a trap for ourselves. When we recognize that this is what we are doing, the first thing to do is drop it. We bring our attention back into ourselves and become quiet. The wrong — or at least the counterproductive — thing to do is to react to our trap building: "Oh no! I'm building a trap!" What happens then? Countertrap number one. Then it is unending trap and countertrap.

Much of what we are reacting to is our feelings and emotions about things. We fail to see that these require a certain discipline. For instance, I have had some experience with Rottweilers. They are wonderful dogs if you discipline them. But if they are in control — and they are perfectly willing to be the boss — then they become a real problem. Likewise, our emotions are completely willing to be in charge if we let them.

If we cannot train ourselves to be free of our reactiveness, which is another word for tensions, we will never attain a deeper awareness of anything. If we cannot rise above the grip of our own desires, we will never be patient and joyful. If we cannot manage our own chemicals and hormones, how will we ever deal with the greater tensions that come our way? We have to give this some thought.

It is a question of taking a stand. If to intensify our inner condition is to compel our lives to reorganize around us, to take a stand is to compel our desires and emotions into support of that endeavor. It is not that we suppress our emotions or abandon our desires; this is not possible, because as long as we have bodies we will have emotions and desires. The question, however, is this: Who will be in charge? Will our emotions, desires, and tensions run us and therefore be a part of our resistance to growing, or will we create a deeper context in which every aspect of our lives plays a role in supporting our process of discovery?

As we explore these things over time we discover something interesting. We find that our strong reactions, such as anger, for example, are all variations on what I call the mantra of stupidity: "What's going to happen to *me*?" This is true of our frustration, resentment, doubt, and insecurity, all of which are expressions of fear. Each one represents some form of the assumption that something important to us is either missing or can be taken away from us. They are all, therefore, also expressions of the ego, which is the most contracted form of our awareness. Its main objective is to fulfill the biological imperatives to eat and reproduce.

So we talk instead about tracing our emotions back to their source. This means taking them beyond the mantra of ignorance. We recognize all agitation as a contraction of creative energy, and we use the techniques we learn in our practice to release it and restore it to a state of flow.

To take ourselves through this process is not how most people respond to tension. Indeed, none of this qualifies as what most people consider normal at all. It has nothing to do with living a reactionary life, which is usually one of action, reaction, reaction, and more reaction. Rather, it is a matter of stabilizing ourselves internally in a peaceful, disturbance-free state, full of happiness. We sustain that state of freedom, no matter what, in the context of every kind of potential feedback and tension. When we recognize that a tension is coming up, we determine that we will not get caught in it, and we relax.

None of this is easy. Any strong experience — any tension — is going to speak to what we are not. By this, I mean that I have never had a powerful experience suggest to me that I was utterly wonderful, that I was doing enough, or that my work was complete and I could retire. I think that every such experience, irrespective of the wonder that was also a part of it, awakened in me the recognition of whole other dimensions of work for me to do.

The tensions and pressures brought into our lives by other people speak to us with the voice of God about the need for us to attain a broader view of things. I would go further and say that no matter what form they take, the tensions we experience with others are only one thing: the voice of God speaking to us about our own work. They tell us about the direction that work must take and about the need to move on — not from one place to another, but within ourselves. Not too surprisingly, then, most of the time when God talks it is not all that much fun to listen.

The truth, however, is that the emergence of strong energy is never a negative event. Nor is it ever a problem. We make it into one only when we point it at somebody else.

Better to point it at ourselves instead. If we feel some dissatisfaction or agitation, we want to recognize that our own lack of understanding is the real issue.

Hindsight is everybody's genius, and criticism everybody's great capacity. It takes an extraordinary human being to open within him- or herself and nourish a situation through that openness to it, thus allowing it to breathe, grow, and express from within itself something that goes beyond the limitations of our private wishes. In other words, we allow the situation to have its own life.

The need to do this is unending. Rudi once talked about having a vision in which he saw himself as a water buffalo going round and round a millstone, turning it endlessly. For the moment that the vision endured, he experienced his whole life as nothing but that turning of the stone — the same effort over and over again, day after day.

Through our practice of meditation and our effort to release our tensions, we develop the quiet that allows us to penetrate every illusion and see through every drama. In that quiet we find the strength and stability to rise above and digest all our tensions and to participate ever more fully in the infinitely self-renewing process of Life Itself.

In our spiritual work we are trying to peel away layer upon layer of misunderstanding, tension, and pressure, in order for a deeper level of integration to take place. If on one level we hear conflicting voices within ourselves, on another level we discover that these are only resonances of the one voice that wants to grow and express an authentic life.

The whole of anavopaya has to do with this issue of releasing tensions and rising above a situation. This is what Rudi used to call developing the capacity to think vertically. As we release tensions, the energy within us should rise. As we let go of our attachment to a particular concept or form of functioning, the energy is then free to rise and give us a new and higher vision of how things could be. This new vision provides us with a sense of the direction in which we can move.

This is simple, but not easy. We find that we have to repeat this process many times to allow the situation to fulfill itself. If we bring a set of mental, emotional, and hormonal issues to these moments, all we end up with are skewed programs. Still, we can train ourselves to approach every situation by going beyond these more limited issues. In any challenging situation we must cultivate the ability to think vertically, rising above the event and allowing its chemistry to work itself out. Eventually this becomes something that should take us about five minutes to deal with in any given situation.

What it means is that we must simply release everything into the depth of our awareness of the dynamic stillness within us. We have to accept our lives as they are, and respond to them with genuine love and appreciation — even when we are not sure just what they are or where they are going. It is not our job to have to know these things. It *is* our job to establish ourselves in our own inner state and respond from that as called upon, to nourish and support the changes and transformations that are trying to happen in those with whom we share our lives.

This makes it ever more necessary for us to develop our understanding of what I talk about as surrender. This does not mean giving up in the face of our tensions but rising above them. The trick to this lies not in ignoring or repressing anything but in not getting entangled in it, even as we are relating to it. Instead, we release the tension within ourselves at the same time as we bring a creative flow into the event and allow all the tensions therein to dissolve.

Rudi pounded on this idea of transcending tension. He talked constantly about opening and taking our energy deeper. He used to say that it doesn't matter what our excuses or defenses are. Each of us is presented with life challenges that are there for us to get over. Understanding comes only when our experience is based on a flow and on our own effort. This is because when we can transcend and dissolve a particular tension we are no longer bound by its particular pattern.

This means being light and simple. The alternative is being caught up in attachment and density, tension and problems, unfulfilled desires and unrealized expectations, pain and suffering, sadness and sorrow — it goes on and on like this.

Transcendence is lightness and simplicity, openness and under-standing, and not the old refrain "Loves me, loves me not."

Openness — another word for surrender — is what allows us to respond and move spontaneously. Even as we plan and cultivate some sense of direction, we are also able to take surprise events and build on them. We can then be open to the logic trying to articulate itself within us, and to whatever feedback we get. When we can get above the tensions within ourselves and stay there, then nobody can bring us down. In that state, our presence in the life of another person can be a real service.

. . . Allowing the Creative Energy to Flow: Service

Fundamentally, our practice has two aspects to it. One involves refining our awareness of the internal flow; the other, our awareness of the flow that we extend. This we can also call service. Service, or giving of ourselves, is part of anavo-paya. It is a necessary part that broadens us in the process of becoming a big person.

To build into ourselves the willingness to serve carries us beyond the patterns by which we are accustomed to living. It enables us to respond with some genuineness and to bring a sense of the quality of Presence into whatever situations present themselves in our lives. It is this willingness to serve that keeps us growing and open to new material.

The responsibility for doing this work falls on us. We should always be ready and willing to demonstrate our under-standing of our practice and how it must be articulated in the world. It must be something we can communicate right now to anybody in concrete and practical ways. If we cannot do this, then we are actually communicating that a person who has practiced meditation doesn't have to do anything real with it. This is never the case. If we are not careful to manage this situation well, it becomes one of the ways we can seriously undermine our inner work.

We have to learn ourselves that if we are not willing to do the shit jobs, we will never be allowed to do the more creative ones. This is true anywhere. When we see an opportunity to serve the situation going on around us, rather than thinking it beneath us, we have to take it as an opportunity. This doesn't exactly mean we have to reach out to it, but within ourselves we have to be open and allow ourselves to flow in whatever way presents itself. We cannot be afraid to extend ourselves.

I think Rudi appreciated me not because I was the flashiest person there — I was probably a serious hick — but because I performed. I understood that this was what I was there to do. I was not there to look good or get a lot of attention and recognition. I was there to function, because it is through our ability to perform that we learn, which is another way of saying that we learn by doing. So, Rudi had to explain very little to me.

The point of service is to give of ourselves for contact with a totally open system, and thereby endlessly to learn and experience transformation. This has nothing to do with any "other" in the way that we usually think, because the bottom line is that there is no real other. If there is only one thing, then even when we love something that appears to be other, we are also loving ourselves. In truth, all of it is ultimately love of the Self and speaks to the unity of Self and other.

So in a way, service has nothing to do with altruism at all. We may hope that others find it meaningful and valuable, but we do it to know what is in our own souls. In this sense service becomes an expression of our love of Life Itself. A life of service becomes possible because of our experience, through practice, of our own infinite resource. It is the way we extend our limits and appreciate that resource, the pulsation of Life. We release ourselves into the moment and thereby extend and overcome our finitude.

This process is a fusion of internal and external and a subsequent liberation of the individual from any sense of limitation — that is, of circumstance, condition, body, mind, emotions, personal history, ego, desires, delusions, and every other possible finitude. It is because of our dedication to becoming finer people that we begin genuinely to feel and understand the living connection that we share with every other human being. This is love. We will see it come up powerfully at different times. Sometimes it will be in the form of a person, sometimes as an experience or a phenomenon. We will see it at work, and we will understand it.

Out of our awareness of the flow and the fluctuation of our awareness from one thing to another, finally we recognize that underlying this exchange is a total unity. I suppose this in itself is a powerful argument for learning to love everything. As we learn how to love we become open systems, releasing from within ourselves the potential for extraordinary transformation.

At the same time — and here is the paradox — our service has nothing to do with binding us to other people. It is not a tacky deal. Instead, we free ourselves from that stickiness by releasing all our concepts about what it is supposed to be. For that matter, any time we get too analytical about this event, we invariably cause a constriction to take place in it. We simply have to free ourselves from too much speculation about it and just be natural. When it is there to take, we take, not worrying about it too much. When we have something to give, we give, without worrying too much about that either. This is what keeps the whole process alive and functioning.

Nor do we need to know in advance how anything will turn out. People sometimes wonder whether the act of service requires a great deal of discrimination. Not really. This may seem contradictory, but it is not. It is true that after a while we develop a certain capacity for discrimination, but in the beginning we just start wherever we are. Otherwise we set up a condition in which we will never serve, because the perfect moment will never be there.

The appropriate precondition will never come into being. If we wait for it to do so, we give ourselves the perfect excuse: Well, I would have if I could have, but it just never happened." This is really nothing but a variation on the mantra of ignorance: "What will happen to me if I extend myself in this way? What might I lose? What will they give *me*?" Better to simply *do*, and discover from the doing. Talk, after all, is one of the cheapest things there is.

It takes time to internalize this approach to our lives, and as I said earlier, we will inevitably make mistakes in the process.

I have not met anybody who has not. But this is fine, because it is our mistakes that teach us what we don't want to be like and what is not right. We thereby learn to cut through the details and get to the point where we have some sense of what is right and true. There is no problem with making even a lot of mistakes as we learn this. They are not all that expensive, unless they cause us to close our hearts. Even then, that happens only at our expense.

I have the same feeling about the mistakes I have made. Of course, I have improved some — I now only make about six a day. But one of the main things I have learned about mistakes is that you don't shoot yourself when you make one. There is a larger mistake beyond making a mistake, and that is beating yourself over the whole event. What you do instead is not to repeat any given mistake more than three or four times.

I cannot emphasize enough that for us to do this we must have a lifetime commitment to growing. There can be nothing in our lives that we can be satisfied we know enough about. This requires that we develop some specialization, choosing something that interests us and immersing ourselves in that. We then extend that capacity for quality into every other field of our lives, since all fields ultimately interact.

The mechanism by which we do this is called service. As a training mechanism, service plays an important part in our development. After that, however, it goes beyond being such a mechanism and becomes a lifestyle.

As we become more adept at maintaining our balance, we promote balance through the whole field to which we are relating. Conversely, when we are out of balance, we only disturb the field — at which point it reaches out, whacks us, and keeps on whacking us until we reach some new level of inner equilibrium.

The experience of the energy *is* balance and harmony. They are the same thing. One is experiential; the other, a cognitive awareness of it. We establish ourselves in that condition as our whole existence is transformed into an act of service permeated with wisdom and understanding. This happens naturally in the course of our practice.

As that natural condition emerges, our minds cease to wander and we experience samadhi. There is nothing to destabilize us, nothing we want or do not want. Instead, we remain aware of all the activities in which we engage on a daily basis, even as we experience the inner dynamic stillness of our own creative potential.

The Shifts

*It takes some consciousness to lower resistance when we
wish to surrender. The deeper your insecurity, the stronger
the resistance; the greater the ego, the stronger the resistance. . . . To gain life you have to surrender life. In this
sense, the more alive you are the faster you will grow.*

— RUDI

Any time we set about learning something, we have to
go through a process of mastering the mechanisms — of
learning a new kind of language. This is true whether we are
beginning to play an instrument or learning to operate a com-
puter program. Every activity has its own terms and techniques that we must first learn, then practice, before we can
feel at ease with them. This takes work and effort.

As we saw in our discussion of anavopaya, what characterizes the experience of the beginning student is the emphasis
on work and individual effort. We work to get the attention
of the teacher and to develop some kind of relationship with
him or her; we struggle to master technique and to feel some
kind of a flow; and we make the effort to extend ourselves in
service to those around us. We begin to realize that we have a

choice in how we respond to tension, and that what we choose has a big effect on how we experience any event in our lives.

We can continue at this level of work indefinitely and draw real benefit from it in the process. But if we really care about growing as human beings, our work has to go deeper. Otherwise at some point we are going to feel we are only struggling with variations on the same questions and issues over and over again. It is the intensity of our longing to grow that will lift us out of this.

This process, in itself, is not easy, and we will encounter all kinds of internal resistance. The ego, for example, finds ten thousand ways to scream and whisper the perennial mantra of ignorance, "But what's going to happen to *me?*" This, ultimately, is always the biggest challenge to our growth, because even though the forms this question assumes look different and feel important in the moment, the bottom line is that they all have the same effect.

The ego takes the energy that was about to generate real growth within us and diverts it back into shoring up the ways of thinking and feeling with which we are already familiar. This is because the ego is less than fond of change. So whenever we find ourselves wrestling with something, the chances are good that some aspect of the ego is at stake. All the turmoil we go through may make us think we have changed, but we have not. Instead, we have only dug ourselves more deeply back into the pit of the familiar.

However, if we are really attuned to the process happening within us, we will understand these ups and downs for what they are — shifts in our awareness as our practice brings about the rewiring of our whole system. When we can understand that this is what is going on, we are able to open our hearts to these shifts and allow them to work themselves through us.

Three shifts in particular can arise to challenge us. The first is the tendency to misunderstand what we mean by growing. This can lead us to work harder and harder in ways that repeatedly externalize our energy. This continues until our understanding shifts and we recognize that the effort required in spiritual work has nothing to do with working harder and harder, but only with letting go of effort and struggle — that is, with surrender.

Second, we will confront many doubts and fears, some of which will shake and disturb us profoundly. Here the ego has a major field day. The issue in this case is the shift from doubt to trust. Third — and this is yet another step in deepening our wish to grow — we realize that we must concentrate and intensify this wish into a one-pointed focus on growing. We must do so to the degree that this focus underlies and orients every one of our undertakings. This one-pointed focus is what we call commitment. So this is the shift from wish to commitment.

Each of these three shifts challenges us with the option of getting stuck, or of entering more fully into our spiritual work. This makes us, as the political activist Eldridge Cleaver used to put it, either part of the problem or part of the solution. This must be so, since we are the ones who choose, and because there is no avoiding the choice. Even when we keep on doing what we have always done, and getting what we have always gotten from it, we are still making a choice. Ultimately the issue is always the same: How deeply do we want to grow?

FROM STRUGGLE TO SURRENDER

The word "surrender" as it is used in relation to spiritual development does not have the negative connotation it often has in ordinary speech. The act of surrender, as the term is used here, is the voluntary casting off of the thoughts and emotions that interfere with the realization of the spirit within. There is often a sense of buoyancy or floating — it is a freeing of oneself from the dimension of the earth. Something within is returning to a level on which it belongs.

— RUDI

The "Work Harder" Approach

Many of us start spiritual work because we want to improve our lives. Generally we are interested in alleviating some set of circumstances, problems, or symptoms we have been experiencing. Maybe we don't want to be lonely; maybe we don't want to be broke. Maybe we are tired of feeling pushed around. Whatever the particulars, what we are usually looking for is a greater sense of control over our lives. So to one degree or another we start spiritual work with some interest in gaining more power over these events, and in using this power to awaken new possibilities and choices for our self-expression. We figure that a spiritual practice just might help us do this.

In the process of learning the basic elements of our practice, we begin learning to dissolve our tensions and release a flow of energy within ourselves. As a result, we may find our individual lives becoming revitalized, our health problems resolving, and much of our psychological distress being alleviated. As we have more of our creative energy available to us, we find ourselves drawn to invest that energy in all kinds of activities. We may go back to school, pursue new career options, get involved in new relationships or improve ongoing ones, or undertake any number of other externally oriented projects. As our lives unfold in these ways, we have the definite experience of what we usually think of as growing.

When this happens, we start to get hold of the fact that we have more real choices than we thought. We discover we can do things to change our chemistry, our minds, and our feelings. As we practice doing this and even have some success at it, it feels pretty good. So we go along doing the same thing.

At some point, however, we may experience what feels like a decline in our practice, as though we are somehow retreating from our spiritual work. At best this may make us feel guilty; at worst we may decide we are some kind of failure. So, we decide that the remedy must lie in working harder at it. We tell ourselves, "I just have to try harder and make more of an effort." We may also feel we are somehow doing the whole thing wrong, so we think about how to change our approach. This makes us work even harder still as we try to do everything right.

There are three problems built into this "work harder" approach. The first is that it sets off a kind of crisis orientation within us. It denies the reality that falloffs are just another part of the pulsation of Life Itself. Every event starts out as one thing, becomes something else, and then becomes something else again. As this happens, all the various energies within it come to the forefront, including pauses and falloffs. This is just as true of our spiritual work as it is of any other part of our experience.

All the breathing and practicing, working and toiling, and churning and burning we do is going to alter our systems on every level. So it is natural that we get to points where we feel stuck. Then one of two things will happen. A shortsighted person will say, "I'm doing all this work and seem to be getting nowhere. I'm tired of it, and I can't do it any more. This whole spiritual thing must be wrong because it doesn't work. These people don't know what they're doing, and what is that guy bothering me for, anyway?"

A reaction like this says a lot about a person's expectations, which brings us to the second problem with the "work harder" approach. Many people enter the process of spiritual work with some preconceived notion of what they are going to discover. When they don't discover *that*, they get disappointed, quit, and go back to searching. A person with some vision, on the other hand, will say, "Maybe my understanding and my expectations were a little bent in the first place. In fact, maybe I ought to re-think my assumptions about the whole thing."

Most of us are conditioned to want some concrete measure of whether or not we are successful in what we are doing. It is not too surprising, therefore, if we enter our inner work with the idea that there will be some system of merit badges to indicate whether or not we are making progress. We may expect a lot of bells, whistles, and bright lights to go off as proof of some kind of spiritual accomplishment.

All of this is beside the point. You can see Tibetans landing in spaceships, and not have grown in the least as a human being. For that matter, there are infinite ways a person can manifest real growth. We may think that working harder in our practice has something to do with finding "the right way" to deepen our awareness. Just what, however, *is* "the right way?" For every person it is somewhat different. Even if we didn't end up with a hundred variations, we would still have at least some twenty or so major themes.

It is like asking how many different theories of good government there are. All such cultural and logical pathways of self-assessment have little meaning when we are talking about infinity. How, then, can we sit down to evaluate the whole experience and say, "I am a success at this," or "I am a failure"? These questions are meaningful only if we are looking for sustenance in the moment, and not for a deeper freedom and sense of total well-being in the long run.

Usually, working harder is our response to feeling that we are inadequate in some way. It is therefore generally not the appropriate place to start. It is not even what we want to focus on in the first place. Rather, we want to focus directly on becoming attuned to the rhythm of whatever system we have chosen to stabilize ourselves in.

As an analogy, suppose we are in school and find ourselves falling behind in our studies. Usually this makes us decide we have to work harder, which seems a natural enough assumption. Even so, it may not be the best strategy for doing well over the long haul. In the course of that exaggerated effort, we create more tension. It becomes harder than ever to take in information and therefore we do not absorb things as rapidly. We notice we are falling further and further behind, and we start to get tired. Our resistance increases, so we try to make ourselves work that much harder. As long as the process follows this logic, there is no end to it. All we end up in is a nosedive.

We want to avoid engaging in approaches that will only make us more tense and nervous. Overreacting to anything is only self-defeating. The best thing is to maintain a steady, disciplined approach, doing something every day and keeping it light and simple. The point is that our ordinary psychological responses to chaos and change, as well as all our judgments about success and failure, are simply not relevant to this kind of inner work. What *is* relevant is our capacity to maintain our balance and keep ourselves oriented toward the fundamental rhythm of the larger field of creative energy. We do this by sustaining the simple discipline of our practice.

Growing Is Not About Control

The third problem with the "work harder" approach is that it grows out of the assumption that if we just work hard enough, we can control the outcomes in our lives. Yet not one of us has any real degree of control over how our lives are going to work out. We may delude ourselves into thinking we can control something, but it is really not possible. This carries over into our expectations about our inner work. To grow is to give up even these expectations and become increasingly comfortable with the total uncertainty of Life Itself.

Growing is not about having more control over the events in our lives or over the results of our inner work. A real spiritual practice involves learning to have the kind of inner balance that enables us to move into areas that would otherwise cause us to panic, without panicking. It trains us to keep that balance as we refine our awareness of the pulsation of Life present in all our experience.

When we can do this, we find that we can proceed slowly, with our attention on the values we are trying to express and an attitude befitting the circumstances. We move through them, full of awareness as to why we are there and what we are doing. Then we get to work and become connected to the situation, forgetting about whatever insecurity we felt in the beginning. We start unfolding whatever is there for us to do. Either that or we say, "Well, this is one of those things I can afford to keep moving right on through." It is that simple.

When we relinquish our need for struggle and for getting control, we also become more open to all kinds of unforeseeable possibilities. This is a profound release. We discover that our practice has nothing to do with controlling our environment but only with mastering ourselves. Moreover, if we examine the question of control with some care, we come to the conclusion that we are never in control and that the whole notion of control itself is an illusion. The same thing holds true for security. If we try to buy some, we quickly discover it is not for sale. Control and security go together, and neither exists.

But there is an even more subtle issue here. As we recognize that we are much more than our bodies and minds, we encounter something that goes beyond either one — some spirit within us that is fundamentally and essentially the biggest part of us. Although it permeates our minds, thoughts, and desires, it also goes beyond all this worldly business. This spirit is the essence of who we are. At the same time, we are not its full expression. That is, *it* is not limited by what we are.

This spirit, this power of Life Itself, is in charge. *It* moves whatever happens in our lives, however much we struggle or fight to keep it from happening. As we allow our creative energy to flow and look carefully at what happens in the process, we begin to see that it is the power of the spirit within us. Moreover, we begin to understand that it is the spirit that is in control. As we watch for a while how this spirit unfolds itself and how it works, we cannot help but be dazzled by its subtlety, elegance, and grace. We see that it works much better than our minds do, and that its scope and capacity are much greater than our own physical power or anybody's intellectual ability.

Having observed this for a while, we stop struggling and start to trust it. We understand that our efforts to work harder are circumscribed by the capacities of our bodies, minds, and emotions, and that these are pretty limited places from which to start. We cease to insist on going this way or that, and just relax. In doing so, we have done something that is extremely difficult for most people: We have admitted to ourselves that we don't know whether we are going to win or lose, but we recognize that, either way, life goes on. We acknowledge that we can live through whatever happens.

The funny thing is that once we let go of our concern about success and failure, winning and losing, or any other kind of control, something starts to enable us to sense the distinction between the two. Then we find we can just skip most of the losing. Our intuition is never perfect, but it is greatly heightened. Because we have inner security, strength, and happiness that are not contingent on money, sex, power, or anything else in the world, we become increasingly free of these things. Then we can enjoy whatever happens to us.

Working harder at anything is an elusive issue because, as it turns out, it is never so much a matter of how hard we work as how much time we spend actually paying attention. In our practice, for example, the real idea is for us to develop the ability to sustain our concentration for long periods of time. It takes practice to develop that deep attunement, and at that stage the notion of effort becomes much more subtle. Indeed, some of the more obvious forms of effort can even operate as obstructions.

So we want to be at once relaxed and alert all the time. This is what yoga training is about. As Rudi used to say, "The outside should be calm like the surface of a lake on a windless day, while the inside should be like a furnace." The inside should be ablaze with the fire of divine love all the time.

Not of Our Doing

Each of us has two choices as we move through life in our many ways. The first is to take inventory and be disappointed. In fact, if we do so, we invariably *will* be disappointed, because we can never have enough of finite things to satisfy us fully. The material aspects of our lives are all sucked away from us over time, just as our relationships come and go on their way. Throughout all of this we can choose a more refined understanding and experience of the evolution that can take place within us through our inner work. This is the second choice. When we can do this, we begin to appreciate the nature of all experience and recognize what is valuable about life. The process of developing this understanding and attending to what is truly valuable is what establishes us as advanced students.

Despite much of what we have learned over the course of our lives, our real work — growing, if you will — is not about becoming successful or qualified in the physical world. It is not about getting what we want or setting ourselves up in a stable financial situation. It is not about going from being confused, broken people who are emotional wrecks to establishing ourselves as disciplined, mentally well-organized, successful people with an appropriate appreciation of our emotional resources and the capacity for strong, healthy relationships. This is not what I mean when I talk about growing as a human being.

I do not mean there is anything wrong with these things. I, myself, like being in the company of basically healthy and happy people. It is important for us to get good educations, develop careers in the world, and do our work carefully and seriously. This will relieve us of financial stress and will give us a basic sense of competence and confidence in our own abilities. It is also important that we learn to interact with others in more honest and effective ways. Spiritual work has nothing to do with evading life in the real world. Rudi used to say that you cannot escape anything if you are really working.

We are concerned with developing the one-pointed concentration necessary to being engaged in various worldly involvements without their being detrimental to our spiritual practice. Indeed a spiritual practice should, to some degree, develop in us the capacity to deal with the material world. At the same time, the ability to do this, in and of itself, is no necessary indication of our spiritual growth. Nor is it what our work is about.

Only when we have both understood and experienced the limitation of worldly rewards and of trying to use spirituality for gain in the world — otherwise known as spiritual materialism — do we make a true leap of awareness. Sooner or later a person who is going to grow spiritually must recognize that there has to be something deeper in life. So we could say that what we pursue has to shift, including the idea of pursuing anything at all.

What does this mean? From the point of view of our infinite Self, there is no aspect of our manifestation that is in any way imperfect. In a sense, it is only when we cease to struggle with what we *are* that we liberate ourselves to become what we might be. Working harder can never bring us to where we hope to go because at a certain point working harder itself becomes an obstacle. It perpetuates the notion that there is some subtle state other than our own to be sought and acquired. Ultimately, this only gets in our way, because it arises from the perspective that there is an "I" and some "other" in the first place, which is otherwise known as dualistic thinking.

The problem lies in thinking that what we are looking for is elsewhere, or even that we need to *attain* something in the first place. This is true even though as beginning students we use a certain amount of dualistic language in talking about the process. For example, we hear that a person has to attain this, and work for that, and feel something, and so on. For beginning students it is necessary to think like this. Otherwise, when we hear that we are to live happily just as we are, we are likely to make the mistake of assuming that our current state, our actual level of skill, and our ongoing justifications for how we do things are all appropriate — none of which is the case.

No amount of effort on our part will change us, as long as we remain within our original pattern of understanding. To think it will is a little bit like learning to swim in a pool with about a foot of water in it. We develop a whole style based on the water being only a foot deep. The harder we try to swim fast, the less we are actually going to be swimming at all.

On the other hand if we put more water in the pool things happen differently. Similarly our inner work injects more energy into our systems and it is this energy that brings about the changes we experience. Even so, as beginning students we are still probably going to work like mad, thinking, "Hey, I'm making a lot of progress, and isn't it great! This really works and now I'm getting someplace."

It is natural, although egotistical, for us to think this way. Somebody who is a little more observant is going to look around the pool and notice that the level of the water has changed — that the bottom is a lot further away than it was in the beginning. Such a person will notice that it was not his or her own doing at all and will say, "I didn't do anything; the water level changed." This is the point of view of the advanced student.

In recognizing that it was not our doing, we experience a certain release, because we were secretly wondering about it in the first place — did we really do anything differently, or were we just taking credit for the fact that things became different? The observant person is going to breathe a sigh of relief and surrender the need to control anything. This surrender releases the issue of egotism, allowing us to live within ourselves. It opens us to the flow of Life Itself within and around us, and allows us to participate simply and quietly in the unfoldment of that matrix of vitality.

From Struggle to Surrender

In the world the only real chance we have of going beyond struggle and effort is self-awareness. This is the power that enables us to recognize where we have already been and prevents us from traveling the same roads. In other words, self-awareness is the power that keeps us from making the same mistakes over and over again. It is not something for which we have to search because it is already within us. We do not have too little, nor is there such a thing as having too much.

Our cultivation of this self-awareness enables us to make choices that extend our access to a state of inner well-being and promote that atmosphere within and around us. It is what enables this inner mechanism to function all the time, allowing our minds to turn quite naturally, and become witnesses to the highest creative process as it functions within us. This is a matter of working with awareness and of sustaining that awareness as we move through every day. If we can do that, then even when we have to move quickly we do not get lost in the process.

Struggle and toil go to struggle and toil, while awareness goes to awareness. The fire of intense awareness, by its presence, is what transforms us. Having a sense of our energy and feeling it within ourselves allows us to move, speak, and do in a different way. It allows the thoughts within us to happen *from* our awareness of that flow, and changes the nature of our experience. Slowly we begin to see the presence of God everywhere in our lives because, as we simultaneously relax and become more vigilant, a support and guidance unfolds from within us. This grace of God is what reveals to us the unity of all experience.

As long as we are trying to accumulate *things*, whether these be material possessions, relationships, or even some kind of spiritual capital that we think will help us *get* material possessions, relationships, or some kind of enlightenment, all we really accumulate are reflections of our own limited ideas. It is necessary for us to let go of every ambition, to release our emotional expectations and all our spiritual aspirations. This is because ambition of any kind, along with the struggle it generates, is one of the major elements that will complicate our ability to sustain ourselves as advanced students.

Self-realization is nothing other than the recognition of our innate, infinite inner Self. It is a growing awareness of the energy of Life Itself, of spanda, within our lives. All the patterns and forms we experience as attachments obstruct the flow of this realization. If I were to put this whole discussion in a nutshell, I would say that what we have to give up is struggle itself. This is a major step in the process of understanding surrender.

This shift in our inner work is the natural and necessary culmination of our effort as beginning students. Indeed, we must pass through this experience if we are to develop the awareness and the focus that characterize shaktopaya — the awareness of the energy. Otherwise we continue to struggle, looking for solutions in the people, places, and things around us.

At that point we arrive at an entirely different understanding of the word "surrender." Surrender has nothing to do with struggle. It is the process by which, initially, we experience ourselves as breaking up and dissolving in the fire of our awareness. We surrender the limits established by our egos, we surrender struggle, we surrender control. We let go of our ambitions, desires, and fears. It is the daily release of our wants, needs, and fears that allows us the opportunity to participate in a state of unconditional happiness, a state we achieve by the power of self-awareness.

The point of our inner work is to take us beyond struggle of every kind and to bring our awareness of surrender into all our activities. If we cannot bring this awareness into every aspect of our lives, we are only going through the illusion of surrender; real surrender happens when we let go of everything on all levels of our existence.

Suddenly we are looking at something that has always been present; we simply didn't know it was so amazing or powerful. We had no idea we were sitting right next to something that went beyond every concept of "beyond." Then it is not that our effort is less but that the element of struggle in the effort has dissolved. There remains only a progressive attention to detail that causes us to develop a fine and deep understanding, and a growing awareness that all things are expressions of the energy of Life Itself.

FROM DOUBT TO TRUST

If you are not strong enough to trust the process, you will destroy your connection to Creative Energy. It is the simplest thing in the world. . . . It has to do with letting the nothingness that is creativity flow through our system. Eventually it will dissolve even that system, and we will be free.

— RUDI

The Poison of Doubt

The second of the shifts that must come about in our awareness if we are to continue our work as advanced students is the shift from doubt to trust. Abhinavagupta, the great master of Kashmir Shaivism, said that no matter which phase of practice is foremost in our awareness, doubt can poison the whole experience. This seems odd, in one sense, because the Shaivite teachers of old deliberately created various rituals to arouse every kind of doubt and deep resistance possible in a human being.

These rituals were performed in carefully designated settings in order to put them in a sacred context, but underneath it all they were still calculated to provoke resistance and give rise to doubt. Their aim was not to test whether someone was a qualified person or not — no one got in the door if he or she hadn't already proved that — but rather to give that person the opportunity to get in touch with powerful doubt all at once. This forced the individual to learn to deal with such doubt as an integral part of his or her inner work and to move through it into the experience of openness and trust.

We no longer do this with rituals. In our practice we figure that everyday life will, by itself, force us to face many of these same doubts over time, and will cause us to deal with them. Even so, facing our doubts remains no less an important issue in the process of growing. This is especially true insofar as we experience doubts about our teacher, our practice, or our experience of our inner work.

In the broad scheme of things, doubt is nothing but tension. This particular kind of tension comes about as we consciously or unconsciously set up expectations about the people and events around us. The problem arises when we discover that what we assumed was functioning in one way was actually not happening at all as we imagined. Then, instead of looking at our own projections, we become filled with doubts about the people or events we believe have let us down.

Generally we try to eliminate the discrepancy between our expectations and the actuality by blaming the situation for not corresponding to our expectations. Then we experience an overall sense of contraction. We may even shut down and cease to function as open people. This in turn increases our tension, causes us to doubt all kinds of things even more, and generates a growing sense of frustration, anger, and resentment. Yet these feelings only demonstrate the degree to which we remain trapped in our own hopes and desires.

This happens a lot as we go through the initial phase of releasing tensions. The process forces us to face up to many of our expectations, whether about our practice or about our lives in the world. When this happens the challenge is to refrain from letting doubt become an endless loop. Otherwise we end up running in place forever.

All doubt is based on the underlying assumption that reality consists of not one thing but many. Perceiving all the events in our lives to be separate and distinct, we withdraw from the ones we fear and reach for the ones we imagine will make us happy. Herein lies the trap. Doubt always implies extroversion. As long as we are unaware of our basic unity with the energy of Life and all its expressions, we cannot help but turn outside ourselves to look for happiness and fulfillment. That extroversion then starts to operate as an overall orientation.

When we don't regularly open our hearts and, with a certain degree of enthusiasm, renew our quest for understanding and our examination of ourselves, we invariably find ourselves trapped in a contracted set of expectations. The ego is the source of this confusion because it is what crystallizes our sense of individuality into a set of boundaries that require defending. We end up feeling isolated and alienated — in some way inadequate or incomplete — and, out of this feeling, we spin a web in which we catch ourselves. Our difficulty arises from our lack of perspective about our individuality.

In doing our inner work, we first deepen our awareness of how, in fact, these boundaries are not real. Second, we practice stabilizing ourselves in that awareness. Moreover, we begin to learn that instead of entering a situation with some expectation which is likely to engender a doubt, it is better just to go along carefully and see what happens. Instead of building channels only so wide for our lives to flow through and saying, "My life is going to flow first here, then there, and it has to be just the way I want it," we take down the walls in our heads, open our hearts and minds, and start to see where our lives can go when we let them. Instead of imposing our expectations on our lives we make whatever effort is really necessary and then step back.

This, too, is surrender.

Self-Doubt

Doubt can hit us particularly hard in the form of self-doubt. This is the doubt we have about ourselves as we confront our different desires and feelings of limitation. Such doubt can act as a kind of paralysis, stopping our energy from flowing freely in the different situations we face, so that we find it more and more difficult to do our inner work.

When we get into this loop, we keep thinking there must be something we are missing — some capacity in ourselves, some form of contact with the teacher, some degree of understanding. We get so stuck in thinking about what we must be doing wrong that we forget to do our real inner work. We may even imagine that all this doubt *is* our inner work. It is not. Furthermore, you will notice how neatly this way of getting stuck lends itself to the impulse to work harder, which we discussed in the last chapter.

On the other hand, there is also some risk that self-doubt can become a cheap excuse. "Oh, I can't do this; I'm not good enough." Whenever I hear this, I think of Rudi, who came from a demanding and sometimes even brutal background that gave him no preparation for doing the kind of inner work he did. Rudi himself talked about his various limitations while recognizing at the same time his refusal to be confined by them.

What Rudi brought about in himself always stands for me as an example of the truth that anybody who wants anything need only do the work. There is no work so complicated that it is impossible. What can *feel* complicated is getting ourselves to go beyond our many excuses and simply do it. When we do not, however, self-doubt turns into a basic case of resistance and a justification for not working. Then if we see some area in our lives that needs to be addressed, we fall down in a heap instead of doing something about it.

So when we feel doubts about ourselves, it is better to get up and simply get to work in order to dissolve the tensions from which the doubt arises. This is where the discipline of regular practice that we establish early on in our spiritual work shows up to support us. We just keep on going and discover that self-recrimination has no place in this work. Understand this well: When we experience self-doubt, getting back to our basic inner work is the best response. Moreover, when we can do this, self-doubt may actually even be a positive thing. It doesn't mean we are really incapable but only that we have not flexed our muscles in a particular arena.

When I say we should never doubt ourselves, I would add that there is a difference between self-doubt and humility. Humility is a way of recognizing that we are all capable of acting like complete fools at any time. Once we accept this, it becomes difficult either to be too impressed by or too down on ourselves. We see that our human condition is a joke that we have to learn to laugh at, just as we must learn to laugh at ourselves. This is humility. It is also a part of the process by which we surrender the boundaries of our egos.

So we continue to pay attention to our practice the best we can and keep egotism out of it. How do we do this? To put it at the most basic level, again, we do our own inner work. Then we become better able to see ourselves as we are and we discover that what is there is not so bad. Through practice we find that there is every reason to have faith in the deepest part of ourselves and that everything else is not nearly so important as we thought it was in the first place. This is one reason why we have a teacher: not to get us to "believe" in him or her but to guide us toward trusting that in which the teacher trusts, the power of that inner spirit.

All too often we have only the small picture in mind. Because we are so attached to this, the big picture of the situation escapes us. Yet if Life really is only one thing, then even though we are each a unique manifestation of it, the Life within every individual is also one. If that is true, then we are a part of that one spirit that has given rise to the whole universe.

In this light, to talk about "trusting ourselves" is a somewhat problematic way to put it. I don't trust this body, and I don't trust this personality. Do I believe, for example, that this body, left to its own impulses, will naturally behave at the level of the highest insight? Sure I do — and the check is in the mail. Through our inner work, however, we are able to demonstrate a creative presence in our lives that works perfectly and appropriately so many times that soon we learn to trust in *that*.

Learning that we can trust the creative energy of Life Itself enables us to relax more and more because we know we don't have to make things happen by the force of our will. Rather we recognize that this creative energy attracts all experiences to us and mediates all outcomes. We find that we can relax, attune ourselves to it, and let it work itself out through us. We simply add the right words at the right moment, just to keep things flowing.

Real Trust is Not Blind But Conscious

Any kind of real life depends on learning to go beyond our doubt in order to trust both ourselves and others, because trust, in itself, is also one. The more we trust ourselves, the more we are able to trust others. The more we do that, the more we see both the limits of our own humanity and those of other people. Seeing this, we sidestep potential mis-understandings because we know, in practical terms, what to expect and also what we ourselves are capable of doing.

We cannot be deeply honest people until we have the ability to trust. Without that, what is life except an endless drama of walking around trying to screw somebody else and avoid being screwed? There is, of course, no way any of us can avoid being cheated or let down at one point or another. Things just work that way. But does that mean we go around for the rest of our lives trying to defend ourselves against the experience? Better simply to open our eyes, use our brains, and listen and look with some care. This is the safest way to avoid being let down.

If we expect that our feelings will never get hurt, we are dead meat. Moreover, we will never learn anything about trust. Kahlil Gibran says something like, "When love's wings enfold you, allow it, even though the pinions may prick you and cause you pain." In our relationships with others, if we look and listen carefully, we will naturally come to understand our own creativity, that of others, and the many ways in which both get expressed.

There are always going to be limits to everyone's pro-gram, and sometimes we will get screwed. This doesn't make any of us bad people, nor is it an excuse for us to get angry with anyone else. No judgment is necessary. We can simply take the whole thing as a joke. If we do occasionally fall into someone else's limitations we can just slap ourselves on the back and say, "Boy, that sure was a good one on me." There is no need to say anything else.

Real trust is not blind but conscious. A blind trust means that we allow anyone to walk up to us and say, "Have I got a deal for you!" — and we believe it. Conscious trust is what happens when we can tell the difference between who really does have a deal and who does not. Then we may not buy into it, but we also have no need to become angry with the other person. In other words, a conscious trust implies that we know the limits of what we are dealing with.

When I speak of trust, by the way, I do not mean the four noble trusts such as, "The check is in the mail," and so on. Instead, I am talking about a deeper trust that, in a way, we could call a binding. What do I mean by this? It is a binding *of* love as well as a binding *in* love. This trust will present us over and over again with opportunities to deal with tensions. It will also provide us with the strength, the ground, the understanding, and the support to deal with those tensions. We base our lives on it in an individual sense, and it becomes the doorway through which we ultimately have access to understanding the nature of Life Itself.

Therefore we develop a living contact not with a doctrine, dogma, or the answers provided in credos, but with the power of Life Itself. In this way, we train ourselves to have the kind of discipline over our minds and energy that allows us to experience within ourselves a total trust in the energy of Life, or God.

Trust and Faith

I am sometimes asked whether this total trust is different from what some spiritual traditions refer to as faith. I would say that it is, in this sense: A spiritual search begins with a certain sense of awakening. That awakening is like what happened one day years ago when I went to a museum. On that particular day, for the first time, I actually *saw* a work of art. In a way, this was a simple moment. Yet for me it was quite dramatic, because I had spent an entire summer going from museum to museum all over Europe, looking at everything everywhere and seeing very little of it. When I finally did see it, it was as if someone had opened my eyes. Do you remember the first time you *heard* a piece of music? Of course, it was not the first piece of music you had ever listened to, but that is not the same thing.

Our real spiritual work begins with such an awakening. It is a recognition of the power of Life Itself within us, which has always been there. All along we had been thinking of ourselves as bodies, thoughts, minds, and desires, when suddenly all of that is cut through and we wake up to the fact that we are a purely dynamic event of conscious, creative energy.

To have contact with that energy and recognize it is also the beginning of our understanding of trust as something we experience in a palpable way. That is, we feel the thing we trust because it is really there. Whether or not we want to accept it into our lives and deal with it is our own challenge. Whether we do so or not does not change the fact that it is still there. As we open our eyes to what we are, our spiritual work becomes a question of learning to trust it. This is the intermediate stage of renewal.

I do not usually use the word "faith" when talking about our openness to this energy, because the word faith so often implies a response to something unknown and untested. I associate it, for example, with a blind acceptance not founded on prior experience. We believe something just because somebody else in authority has said it is so. In my opinion, any requirement that a person accept something without real experience to back it up is absurd, not to mention potentially dangerous.

But if we *were* to talk about faith, I would say that authentic faith should be based on something that has been demonstrated. Real faith involves having confidence in something that, from experience, we know works. We have seen it do so over and over again. Then we don't have to waste a lot of time testing it out one time after another. To the extent that this is so, we could say that faith and trust are the same thing.

Whether we talk about faith or trust, it is not going to make the actual experience any easier to understand. When we are talking about spiritual subjects, we may vary our language and analogies in order to walk around the whole thing and see it from a number of different vantage points. We may find that some of these intersect to give rise to new insight. Nevertheless, the words themselves can never fully articulate the essence of this, because it is unexplainable. Words cannot encompass it; they can only reflect it dimly. It is experience that makes the difference.

Resolving to Trust

This process is one of those things that doesn't seem to have any exact beginning but is, instead, something of an endless loop. To be able to trust, we have to have some experience of it in the first place. Yet to have that experience, we have to have some idea of how to do it, which brings us to the edge of a cliff. So at some stage we simply resolve to trust. If we happen to hit the ground a couple of times, we dust ourselves off and understand not that trust is a terrible thing but that maybe we have not learned everything there is to know about it. Then we start again.

We learn to trust by trusting. In the process we see both *that* it works and *how* it works. At many points in our lives we come upon situations where our physical, material, and intellectual resources cannot match the challenges we face, where the challenge is so far beyond us that there is nothing to say about it. At the same time, there is also no avoiding what confronts us. In such moments, if we really trust, Life has a way of revealing within us every resource that is required. This is part of what we mean by "surrender." When we give up our limited understanding of what we are and choose instead to trust, we actually give up nothing. We only gain an expanded understanding of the inner Self.

Basically, there are two kinds of life: a life of struggle, which is life as most people experience it, and a life of trust, which allows for infinite growth and permanent happiness. We get to choose which we will live — this is the arena of our free will. It has nothing to do with any kind of intellectual teaching or understanding, or even with any system of yoga. This is a yoga of trust in God, of union in God. It is the release of our attachment to external things and even to any understanding we have of ourselves as individuals.

To bring about this understanding simply takes an open mind and an open heart. It takes the ability to rise above tensions, and to do so without getting entangled in the changes that happen as we release the potential inherent in any given moment. Even though such change is rarely comfortable, our trust enables us to see beyond what is immediate and expedient. Then what we see in everyone concerned are not patterns of limitation but creative patterns through which Life articulates its true nature.

How does this affect our understanding of ourselves as individuals? After all it is the ego that structures our doubts even as it structures our boundaries as individuals. As our sense of trust in life grows, the ego does not actually wane. Indeed, insofar as it has the ongoing function of sustaining our biological integrity, it is not a problem as long as it doesn't dominate our whole system and become the limit of our horizons. We do, however, have an increasingly different experience of our inner resources, which makes the ego less and less dominant as we feel less and less need to hold on to anything.

Only when we trust Life Itself can we accept what it is trying to tell us about its own nature. If we don't trust it, how can we listen to what it says or accept what we hear? How can we allow it to change us and enable us to rise above all our doubts and fears? No matter what we aspire to in this life, and even if we don't particularly care about spiritual work at all, this question of trust is still central to our existence and worth our careful attention. At the very least it will free us from self-pity and fear and from our resistance. At its best, trust elevates us above pain and allows our lives to be unbroken expressions of the joy that is the essence of our intimate experience of the divine.

FROM WISH TO COMMITMENT

My wish is to grow, my wish is only to grow, and what-
ever else happens can happen.

— RUDI

The Wish to Grow

We have talked about the shift from working harder to surrender, and from doubt to trust. The third shift that must come about if we are to go on in our work as advanced students involves the transforming of our general wish to grow into a one-pointed focus on growing. This one-pointed focus we call commitment.

Every human being, to a great degree, is motivated by the experience of a deep inner longing. Paradoxically, most of our activities as human beings represent the effort to mask that longing. We go into our activities and relationships thinking they will satisfy us. In the process we pour our energy out of ourselves in ways that can only undermine our inner work.

Whenever we externalize that longing and pursue something external, we have taken a powerful feeling and allowed it to crystallize into a course of action. Once it becomes behavior, we may even get some positive feedback from it. In the long term, however, we find that the real thing we wanted has somehow eluded us and we have lost our balance. The mind is no help here. It goes this way and that, that way and this. We have a flock of chickens running around between our ears and we don't even know it. Whatever real choices we have to make in the process have nothing to do with anything outside us. Nor are they something we can think our way through. Rather they are resolved by our dedication to a process of inner work.

The heart of this process is the conviction that we want to know the power that supports our lives. This is what we are really expressing when we say we sincerely want to grow as human beings. Our inner work is a tool by which we arouse this power and energy of growth within us. This is an evolutionary, unfolding energy that has within it not just one pattern but the potential for all patterns, so that the possibility of unlimited growth exists within us if we want it. The point is that we have to want it, we have to understand that we want it, and we have to be willing to learn what it means to work at it.

When I lived in Rudi's house in New York, I used to sleep on the floor on an air mattress by the door of the meditation room. I slept under an old fraternity blanket and used my blue jeans as a pillow. Rudi would come downstairs at about five-thirty or six o'clock in the morning. He would look in the meditation room, and I would be waiting there for him. I would jump up, throw on my jeans, and we would go out for a walk. Maybe he would say one or two things to me, but mostly we would walk for an hour in silence. Talking didn't really matter. One day, though, as we were walking along, he just looked at me for a moment. Then he said, "You can't want it one day, not want it the next, and hope to get anywhere." I have never forgotten this.

All growth must start with, and be sustained by, this will to grow. Especially for a beginning person, this is an important thing to cultivate. Consequently, as an initial departure point for people in their practice, I ask them to sit down and take their attention not into their heads but into their hearts, and to ask as deeply and sincerely as they can to surrender and grow spiritually. In your own work you can use whatever language, word sequence, or number of syllables you feel expresses this for you. As you go along in your practice, these details become more important, but at this stage the feeling is everything.

Each one of us comes into this world and tries to create an identity for ourselves. In the midwest, where I grew up, everybody did this by belonging to a fraternity in college. Everybody had his or her own political perspective and social program. These identities that we develop, whatever their form, become the containers into which we fit our lives. We define the boundaries and then circumscribe our understanding of ourselves accordingly.

It is not unlike the dog who goes for a walk and sets out to mark his territory. In this way he is announcing his willingness to stand in defense of that territory against any intruder he can identify. Of course, he is most likely to identify other dogs as threats, so that even though people enter his boundaries along with other creatures, he may not respond on that level at all. This suggests that his territory, or what he thinks of as his identity, is actually porous. It is not a real, absolute boundary, but an illusion of sorts. Is this so different from the way we set up our own lives?

The wish to grow is the foundation upon which we establish a much broader and infinitely more inclusive sense of identity. As we change the feeling — the frequency within ourselves — the crystallization that has established itself as our minds and emotions is going to start to break down. Few of us will take these boundaries down in such a way that they stay down for good; most of us move them out slowly. Still, with practice and work, we can keep extending them indefinitely.

As we practice this wish to grow, we begin to realize that we can go beyond whatever state we are currently in. Put a little differently, we have the capacity to change our own vibration. When we feel angry, sad, depressed, or anything else, instead of getting sucked into that feeling we can take our attention to a deeper place within ourselves. Then every experience becomes reduced to its fundamental essence of pure energy.

Rather than channeling this energy back into the familiar structures and patterns set up by the ego, we allow it to be absorbed within us much more deeply, perhaps even as a very different sense of identity. In this way, every experience can become a positive one instead of serving to reinforce the walls we build that separate us from the love within and around us.

As we slowly take down those walls, we find that we no longer have to dance to the music of anger, depression, ambition, or anything else. Instead, we can learn to dance to a much deeper music that is constantly in balance with the highest, best interest of all of Life. This is called love; it is also surrender.

That we do not concentrate on this intensely all the time is all right. The point is to work at it as best we can. Once we discover that we have a simple tool in our hands that can change our whole lives if we practice with it and use it, then we are likely to become more and more determined to learn about it.

Both Focused and Flowing

I would like to return to the question of intensity for a moment. Rudi used to talk all the time about this process of intensifying the energy through our wish to grow. This process requires a simple, disciplined life in which we continuously orient ourselves toward our inner work. It does not matter whether we are talking about our relationship to pain or pleasure: Both play a part in the process of intensifying our creative energy as it refines our bodies and minds.

Within this general wish to grow, however, there is a point in time where there must be a transition. If we think about spiritual growth and say to ourselves, "I want, I want, I want," and if what we want is not forthcoming according to the measure of how we have defined it, we become disappointed and say, "Well, I didn't get it, so it must not have been there in the first place." This is incorrect, since we do have it all along, and it is always there to get. The real issue is our own appreciation and recognition of it and our willingness to attend to it constantly.

Wanting and having a relationship with another person are two different things. Likewise, wanting and having a relationship with the divine are different, as are wanting to grow and actually growing. When we think about wishing to grow, we generate one kind of feeling. When we think about being committed to growing, we give rise to an entirely different feeling — one that means we take responsibility.

What distinguishes them is a transformation of our awareness in two ways that might seem initially contradictory. On the one hand, we are cultivating a firm mind with a concentrated focus; on the other, an open one. Firmness expresses itself on several levels. Internally, it enables us to stabilize our minds in an awareness of the vitality of Life.

As we express that wish intently over time, however, it becomes more and more subtle until only the intensity of the wish remains. This is what we mean when we say that we become one-pointed. Cultivating and maintaining that intensity of focus is what brings us to the core of our whole endeavor. To put it a little more formally, the intensification of our energy is the vehicle by which we achieve the recognition of our own potential.

This is an important shift, which occurs as we expand and extend the intensity of our wish and let it take us beyond our entanglement in struggle and beyond our doubts and fears. We train ourselves to be one-pointed in this intensity even as we are also completely open to the unfolding of the energy of Life on its own terms.

What we want to do is cultivate a pure, intense awareness that is both focused and flowing at the same time. This represents a total one-pointedness without becoming a constriction. If we are sitting there saying to ourselves, "I wish to grow, I wish to grow, I wish to grow," and getting tighter and tighter as we concentrate everything down into one point, we are only sitting there flubbing our dubs, as my dad used to say. We have to have a one-pointedness that is also a complete openness.

Paradoxically, this firmness, or stability, is necessary if we are to be completely open to — and thus aware of — the vast array of potentiality present before us. The combination of the two is what makes this awareness truly live, because openness is what allows us to respond and move spontaneously. Even as we plan and cultivate some sense of direction, we are also able to take surprise events and build on them. We can then be open to the logic trying to articulate itself within us and to whatever feedback we get.

Otherwise our deep desire to grow can turn into a kind of fanaticism that is firm, but not open in the slightest. It then becomes an intolerance that, ultimately, is a prison for us. On the other side of the coin, both focus and firmness are necessary because an undirected openness can make us completely superficial, having no structure with which to guide our awareness. Then we become like a river without banks, flowing all over the place and getting nowhere. Either of these conditions sets us up to become absorbed by life without absorbing life into ourselves.

Trying to balance commitment and openness at the same time is a delicate matter. If we are open, for example, it may seem as though we have to be open to whatever circumstances flow our way. Essentially, however, the discussion of openness operates on a second level that has nothing to do with anything but the flow of energy. We open to that flow within ourselves. From that openness we recognize the need to promote harmony and balance within our environment through service and the giving of ourselves.

In your own practice you are going to have to learn to bring together the two poles of intense one-pointedness and infinite spaciousness. These have to become part of the same movement. The particular vibration between these poles represents the real refinement of your understanding and attainment. This is the distance between one-pointedness and the ability to release and allow a creative flow to unfold. For some people the distance lies from here to the other side of the planet, making them slow and dull. For others the gap is less. The more the two things coincide, the finer the frequency of our awareness. Thus we want to bring them together. When they converge what we have attained is a profoundly dynamic inner stillness.

Many voices speak within us and motivate us, but these are really only our different tensions talking. Underneath that multiplicity there is one voice. Spiritual work is what intensifies that one voice even as we surrender our finite voice into that infinite one. The competition of the many voices is the chorus of confusion. The one voice is the voice of clarity that extends our field of function infinitely.

We can be certain that the greater the intensity within us, the more powerful the change that will come about. This intensity is not an emotional state. For that matter, there should be a minimum of smoke and dust coming out of it. We learn, instead, to keep our bodies and heads relaxed so that when we encounter passion or intensity, the chemistry of these changes will not disturb our minds or distort our vision.

Habits That Die Hard

There will definitely be times when we encounter a lot of resistance to doing the work necessary for this balance to come about. We will also feel a resistance to changing. This is normal. The boundaries in which we have invested tremendously are not just going to lie down meekly. Such patterns — we can think of them together as the ego — are habits that die hard. We will definitely encounter resistance we will have to work our way through; and it *is* real work.

As we work on this, a kind of purer feeling emerges in our hearts, and all the different energy centers of our bodies start to resonate. Perhaps a sensitive person will even start to feel the lines of force connecting those energy centers. We will experience ourselves not as limited individuals or as a set of desires and emotions but rather as a dynamic energy mechanism. This mechanism has the full potential of the energy to which it has given structure. In other words, it has infinite potential.

In observing the process by which this energy mechanism extends itself, we start to understand and experience our whole external life as integrally connected to our internal life. Eventually we observe that there is no such thing as external anything: All form and feeling are of one essence. *This* process is what I mean when I talk about growing.

This is no denial of worldly life, as far as I am concerned, but we have to have our priorities in order and know what we really want. If, for example, we are intent on the structure and form of the energy, then we may never really know its essence. That is our choice. Likewise, if we want to know the essence, we may have to sacrifice concern for the form. Interestingly, however, in sacrificing our preoccupation with the form, we then encounter a bigger form, then bigger forms beyond that, and so on, until finally we realize the infinite form. It all starts very simply, with the deep wish in our own hearts to grow spiritually.

If we change our own vibration, then we attract two things from our lives: first, many tests of our sincerity and, second, the support to our endeavor. This is natural, because as the structures in which we have invested start to vibrate more, we can expect to feel some internal agitation. However, if we can persist in our endeavor, we increasingly discover an inner resource which is, paradoxically, also the source of our agitation. This supports us in the midst of all the change.

Intensifying our wish into commitment and becoming deeply open at the same time does not happen without some pain. As I have suggested, any process in which we release tensions brings us face to face with our own expectations and desires. This was true, for example, for the Buddha in his own process of awakening. He sat under the tree and said, "I will go no further. I will sit here and not be moved until I finish my work, until I attain realization." He meant it. He spoke with complete conviction and one-pointedness, and within three days realization happened for him.

At the same time, it is said that in those three days every kind of temptation and desire imaginable visited him. This is one way of looking at it. Another way, which I suspect is probably closer to the truth, is that the very power of his commitment started to unravel a whole body of tensions in him. These, in turn, gave rise to every desire he had ever had, which he experienced in the form of temptations. He did not close himself off from these things, but because his commitment was strong and true, he refused to be sidetracked. Finally, these same tensions were released as creative energy. They evaporated, merged into the highest state, and he was free.

Thus our real spiritual practice is, quite simply, a total commitment to experiencing the growth possible for each of us as we pass through the changes that Life Itself naturally brings us.

Deciding What We Are About

Let me make an important distinction here. Commitment of this kind does not cancel out our other commitments. It does not give us an excuse to break or ignore them. Therefore it need pose no threat to our basic life circumstance. Of course, some people in our lives may not see it that way and will have trouble with the idea of a commitment that supercedes what they understand as our commitment to them. They may try to test our resolve, in which case, we will find out where we live. If we are careful, we can probably manage most of these tests and keep all the channels open. Nevertheless, we may occasionally encounter somebody who decides that it is either them or nothing. Then we have to decide.

In one sense, the easiest thing would be to bag the whole program; then everybody would be happy. There comes a point, however, when we realize we cannot do this, no matter how much the other elements in our lives may mean to us. What we also discover in the process is that the biggest obstacle we face is ourselves, especially as we run up against our own ambivalence and resistance toward growing.

The bottom line is that we have to have such a degree of commitment that it elevates us above every narrow concern about relationships, careers, or any of our other desires. Instead, we concentrate all our energy on intensifying our wish to grow. This does not mean that our involvement in work or relationships is not important. It is nice if we can have the things we hope for in our lives. However, these come about best in concert with our careful attention to our practice and our ability to live above the level of tension in our own systems. Moreover, if they do not come about, there is nothing we feel the need to do.

The real point is that commitment has nothing to do with becoming popular or getting a better job; it is not about having a fulfilling career, a satisfying family life, or anything at all. If this statement causes us to feel some alarm, it suggests we are still caught up in thinking of our practice in terms of the material and emotional benefits it will bring us. There is nothing wrong with this, but it does act as an index to tell us what our priorities currently are.

It also has consequences. If we come to a spiritual practice out of any kind of selfishness, we will either fall away or learn to appreciate the power and beauty of Life, and in our appreciation, come to understand it. Our profound commitment enables us to make the shift from the selfishness of desire and the attempt to accumulate spiritual capital on the one hand, to selflessness and the discovery of our infinite resources on the other. Then we no longer even talk about growing, insofar as growth implies the notion of accumulation. At this point we are not accumulating anything but simply discovering what is infinite within us.

At a certain point we have to decide what we are all about and what we are really doing with our lives. When we get clear about this, our other commitments fall into line. If we make growing our first priority, this determination will shape every other choice we make thereafter and will inform how we respond to all our desires. For example, having chosen in favor of harmony and balance, we probably no longer elect to be involved in everything that bobs and weaves around out there. How could we, when what we are involved in is training ourselves to be aware of the stillness at the center?

Therefore, commitment as I am talking about it goes beyond feeling commitment to a spiritual practice. Many people practice. We could even say they are dedicated to their practice and have been for a long time — in some cases, for ten, twenty, or even fifty years. This doesn't necessarily mean they have addressed their fears, doubts, or tensions in any real way. It also doesn't necessarily mean they have taken responsibility for creating an environment within and around themselves that allows them to advance their understanding. Thus a person can practice for years without ever being accounted for.

We have to recognize that we can be around for a hundred thousand years and not get it. Longevity is certainly wonderful, and Rudi talked a lot about its value. It *is* valuable in one sense, and it does show a certain quality in a person. However, if we do not take that longevity and turn it into something living and vital, what is the point? After all, anchors last a long time, as do rocks. So what? Longevity is worth no more than a heap of road apples unless we are aware of what we are doing during all that time. In and of itself, who needs it? Cemeteries are shrines to longevity — people never move out of there. So we are talking, instead, about a longevity that must also be dynamic.

If we do our inner work with depth over time, we discover that it is not really we who are doing the work. Rather it is by the very intensity of our focus that the work just happens. It magnetizes that level of truth within us, making its horizon visible to us. Some change and transformation may appear to take place as the whole event organizes itself to manifest, but then it becomes our job not to get entangled in appearances or to become complicated and resistant. It is our job to stay simple and attuned to the purity of that focus. Then, a wonderful thing happens. Whatever our chosen forms of self-expression — and each of us functions in more than one arena — all of them become demonstrations of the intensity of that focus and of the insight attained therein.

Jelaludin Rumi, whom I consider to be the most extraordinary mystical poet who ever lived, called it "the longing," and thought of it as the vehicle that takes us to God. We could also call it the vehicle that takes us into our hearts. I would say that all the different spiritual practices and philosophies are not only vehicles that put us in touch with that longing, but also expressions of what we experience as that longing matures within us.

The experience of longing and the resolve to grow are intimately interrelated because when we can take the intensity of that longing and channel it back into our wish, we are consciously attuning it to the deepest place within ourselves that seeks fulfillment. This transforms longing from an externalized orientation into a spiritual event in which we actually change the focus of that energy and are uplifted in the process.

Once we focus on developing internally, our longing becomes a different affair operating according to an entirely different dynamic. Rather than attempting to identify a set of objectives in order to fill some void within ourselves, we turn our attention to that inner place, which is also the heart of any sense of inner balance. We start to learn something about our own essence in a process that has profound and powerful consequences. Its effect is the discovery, in a very real way, that we are not what we think we are — not our bodies, minds, emotions, or any of our psychological states — and that life is more subtle and sophisticated than any kind of dualistic thinking can encompass.

The more we relate to the infinite potential within us, the more it starts to sink into our brain just what it really is. Commitment is that process by which we stabilize our minds and emotions, and ultimately our entire awareness, in that awareness. If we do not cultivate that stability within ourselves, how will we ever be able to extend it into our environment and serve what we find there? Instead, all we will spread around us will be our own lack of it. So we commit ourselves for the sake of this ultimate stability.

The commitment to grow that we make to ourselves is a way of rooting our conscious mind, or ordinary awareness, in the deeper vitality that is the essence of what we are. Then meditation is the time we spend every day getting in touch with that part of us that is really alive. This is what we are really about, and have been all along.

One-Pointed Love

I said that commitment is a fixing, or holding, of our attention that involves stabilizing our focus and making our energy one-pointed. The paradox in this connection is that it doesn't particularly matter what we choose as a focus. Why not? Because all commitment, pursued deeply, goes to the same place: If we become truly and deeply one-pointed in our focus, ultimately we become one-pointed on love. Any authentic commitment must mature into love because in commitment there is love, and in love, commitment. In a universal sense, there is nothing else but love, from which commitment arises and into which it subsides.

As our own love and devotion toward growing intensify, we find the capacity to renew ourselves endlessly. Because our commitment is an expression of devotion, it is not hard-edged. Rather it is totally loving. This makes it at once an effort and also effortless. It is work, but it is also simultaneously free of struggle. Furthermore, something done out of real love is naturally one-pointed.

If out of great devotion and love we embrace this understanding, we move yet further toward relinquishing the boundaries of our egos. This process purifies us and refines all aspects of our existence. Its essence is our unshakable participation in the finest part of ourselves, in our own highest freedom and joy.

Eventually we become one-pointed in our love for the creative process of Life Itself. Nor is it love alone, but a love founded on respect. It is an awe, amazement, and wonder before the dazzling creative process that continuously unfolds within and around us. This is respect at its most profound. So we can say that our commitment becomes an act of devotion and respect toward, love for, and love *in* that creative process.

This devotion is not something we do or express for some "other." It is not a matter of exalting anyone or anything else. A person who lives a life of devotion, respect, and love is one who does so for him- or herself. It is a fundamental training by which we develop as people *capable* of devotion.

If we can take up the simple discipline of opening our hearts and minds every day, of feeling the flow of Life within us, and of allowing the joy inherent in that flow to manifest thorough us, then we move through every experience, no matter how great the uncertainty we face, filled with the possibility, nourishment, and wonder that mark authentic participation in our own lives.

Commitment of this kind is a powerful thing. We have seen people whose commitment is deep and authentic who have moved whole societies. If faith moves mountains, commitment rearranges solar systems and galaxies. It is only because of commitment that any human being has ever achieved a great spiritual state, first and foremost because he or she was totally dedicated to this pursuit.

As our wish to grow intensifies into a pure commitment to growing as human beings, we recognize that the Life within us has a logic of its own that *it* is trying to articulate through us. The more we get out of its way and allow it to inform us as *it* wills, the more we find we can trust it, and our doubts and fears dissolve. Thus because of this commitment — this devotion — we understand and master the mysterious process of surrender. Then we see God within ourselves even as we come to see ourselves within God, and God in one another.

Mastering the Basics

Stabilize the mind in the practice of meditation, concentrate the consciousness in the heart-sky; this is liberation.

— NITYANANDA

What It Means to Practice

To be an authentic human being takes real work. As beginning students of spiritual work we have three primary things to keep in mind. The first is to ask ourselves just why we are doing the inner work that makes it possible. The real reason we engage in any spiritual practice is to grow as human beings.

In growing we will have experiences that are not easy to deal with, but this is the point of growing. Any situation in which we can grow will necessarily challenge us. A spiritual practice in particular will challenge us because it is not merely an intellectual exercise.

Ordinarily we are trained to take in material, organize it into patterns, and regurgitate it in one way or another. Some of the more successful people in the world are good test-takers. If a person can take tests well in school and do well on the SATs and GREs, then he or she is rewarded tremendously. If we are really good at it, we become a suit, a person whose identity becomes the professional role he or she plays in life.

A spiritual practice is not like that. Any practice with substance to it is going to challenge us in places within us we didn't even know existed. We didn't know, because our mental and emotional mechanisms are structured to filter them out. Different parts of us that have never been touched or challenged — parts that are deeper than our minds and emotions — start to awaken and stretch. As this happens, we are going to have to remember why we are doing this in the first place. Otherwise we will get lost in the awakening of these tender places.

Practice is about mastering the basics, about laying the foundation for all the rest of our inner work. In achieving mastery in any spiritual discipline, the fundamentals are always the most important thing. In our case these fundamentals, as we have seen, are the breath, chakras, flow, and sense of Presence.

The second thing to remember is what it means to practice. Practice means doing something about it every day. It doesn't have to be a long, intense practice, and the opportunities will vary, but it is important to sit down and do our inner work every single day.

Meditation is basic to this. Nityananda talked about it as a focused concentration, the merging of mind into wisdom, the look within. We bring our minds to perfect one-pointedness, stilling them and drawing them away from an externalized orientation. We make our breath harmonious and ultimately single, as our awareness reaches inside to come in touch with and start to observe the energy of Life Itself. One of the fundamental points of anavopaya is to start to examine that pulsation and, through our examination of it, to have access to the highest vibration. This is the resonance and energy of Life Itself.

If we were to synthesize what practice is for a beginning student, we might say that there is a technique to master that involves learning to pay attention to the flow of energy within us as it goes down the front and up the back. We need to pay constant attention, as well, to the energy going on in what we perceive to be outside of us.

We begin by learning to concentrate on every level, with our senses as well as our minds. Gradually even the simplest actions become expressions of our practice. We find in them the occasions for going beyond the confines of our egos and entering into a deeper experience of our real condition. As our boundaries dissolve, so does everything about us that is closed, rigid, and stuck.

Practice means changing our chemistry. Rudi used to talk about the fairy tale of the child who sees an elf under a mushroom. He grabs it, knowing that if he can hold onto it, the elf will grant his wish. The elf turns into fire, a wild animal, and many other things, until finally he turns back into an elf and grants the boy's wish. This, said Rudi, expressed the importance of sustaining our practice even as our chemistry goes through many changes.

Practice means developing the discipline and skill necessary first to clarify our focus and then to sustain it. This requires a fair degree of self-honesty. All of us have personal stories about how we want to grow. The point is to live them. We are all full of ideals when there is no price to pay — dinner at that fine restaurant is wonderful until the bill comes.

In a broader sense, practice is about dissolving tensions not only as we sit in meditation but also in our daily lives. In the process we transform our relationship to our thoughts, emotions, and desires. We do not seek to restrict these powerful forces at work within us. However, as we increasingly live in the recognition of the energy, our whole relationship to their function and action is transformed.

We learn to sit through the discomfort involved. Any time we bring new tools into an event and start to use them to improve the situation, things go along fine for a while until, all of a sudden, everything has to reorganize to accommodate to the new system. No one likes this much. In ourselves, it is the ego having to give up power. This is not easy to do without a lot of pain.

Yet it is like the practice of homeopathic medicine, the origin of vaccination theory, in which you take a little dose of the poison in order to develop an immunity to it. It is the observation of homeopathy that frequently the remedy for a particular condition will first aggravate the condition before reversing it. This is known as "worse before better." The same is true of our own internal reorganization.

Here is where the regularity of our practice is so important. It creates a pattern in our lives of doing this work. This is critical because otherwise when we most need them we will not have easy access to our inner resources. A spiritual practice is most important when the pressure is on because it is in those times that we must already have a well-established connection to those resources.

These different aspects of practice contribute to dissolving not merely our tensions but our ignorance. This does not mean that we replace one piece of information with another. It is not necessary to *know* anything. Instead, we replace one experience with another as we come to recognize what was present in us already all along: something we have always known without being aware that we knew it.

The important thing is to recognize that the ultimate reality is not beyond us in any way. It is our foundation. If we don't see this, it is because we become so wrapped up in the momentary aspects of our existence that we fail to see the forest for the trees. For the person who recognizes that absolute reality is the core of what he or she is, every delusion about the nature of human experience is transformed.

Maintaining Openness

This brings us to the third thing to keep in mind. This is somewhat more difficult and a little more subtle. I would suggest that the crucial part of the practice of the beginning student is learning to maintain an open mind about *everything*. The point to this is that, generally speaking, as successful test-takers we are deceived into believing we have the answers.

Furthermore, in order to sell ourselves in the world and be materially successful, we have to present a convincing case as to why we are capable people. Even though many times we recognize in our heart of hearts that we may be fudging slightly on our resumes and that our sales jobs may include some snow, we still do our best to defend our positions.

As spiritual people we do not need any answers. In fact, it is to be hoped we will mature and realize that answers have little to do with life. In the meantime, until we get to the point where this idea takes on visceral meaning for us, it is best to try for an open mind and not to jump to rapid conclusions or to judge people and circumstances.

Instead, it is our job to look more deeply into the people and situations we encounter. We can look into them and see what is interesting and positive there. What in that particular situation can we build on? This way our inner work translates both into an understanding and a material reality that will continuously uplift and support us.

To cultivate this kind of openness, we give up our false sense of having control over the events within and around us. This becomes the basis for a more direct experience of the power of Life Itself as it moves through our lives. Because of our attention to it, increasingly we notice its presence; we discover that it is the underlying constant in all our experience.

The openness to Life Itself that we cultivate frees us from a great deal of conditioning and many inherent, and inherited, assumptions. I said that life is not about answers. It *is* about learning to live in the middle of complete uncertainty, and doing so gracefully.

As we recognize the potential within us, we see that it is not goal-oriented. Rather it simply *is* fullness and total well-being. Think of it like this: If you were aware of a total well-being infinitely at the core of your existence, what would your attitude be toward the ups and downs of your life? It should be something of a relief to realize that nothing has to be done to know this well-being except to look within ourselves. This is meditation. It becomes apparent to us through our capacity to be open.

In that inner environment we are free to accept ourselves as we are. We become open to ourselves. As we give up struggling, we see that spiritual growth has nothing to do with becoming anything different from what we are. It has nothing to do with becoming a teacher or a saint. There are stories throughout India about monkeys who, through their devotion, attained the status of gods, just as there are stories of criminal gurus and enlightened low-lifes.

It is therefore difficult to think of this in terms of making ourselves into something other than who we are. Who would we pick? The point is to be ourselves in the fullest sense. We do our work and unfold our own highest potential, none of which has anything at all to do with form.

The difficulty with opening ourselves to the inner richness of who we are is that we have a tendency to think we have to work through one thing or another before we can make a shift. We think we have to have resolved all our issues. The problem is that this never happens, because whatever our issues, each one we resolve only generates more.

What I sometimes refer to as the stream of experience is kept flowing by the idea that there is something else we need to work out. If you happen to buy into the idea of rebirth, an endless round of rebirths is also sustained by that notion as we keep coming back to work out just one more thing. It is only the depth of our commitment to growing that lifts us out of this cycle. This is why it is so important that we go beyond both struggle and doubt, and concentrate our energy into that commitment.

Remaking Our Lives

As our attention becomes increasingly one-pointed and our focus shifts, the structures of our lives also change. The kaleidoscope of the world is presented before us. We have the opportunity to choose what we will identify with and be involved in. This is true every day of our lives. We go into the world and have the opportunity to pick and choose exactly what our lives will be. So we are remaking our lives every single day.

The structure of our lives depends on what we identify with. If we identify with the world, what we unfold is limited by the structures of the world and our program will be set by that environment. We have to invest our energy someplace. Either we invest it in every kind of superficial, fleeting thing, or we invest it inside where it has the ability to bring us a great return.

Only when we do serious inner work do we take the energy out of our conditioning and redirect it in a way that increases our range of mobility. Increasingly we identify with what we discover deep within our own hearts. In the process we find out two things. First, all too often we are tempted in our spiritual work to trade off the long-term for some short-term benefit. There may be times when we feel we are only investing, paying out and paying out.

Think of it this way, however. It took the Japanese only fifteen years to transform their economy. It doesn't take that long to transform a life, but we have to be willing to invest, and we have to be there for the long haul.

Second, it really doesn't matter what anybody else is doing. It doesn't matter what is happening in the state of the economy or the body politic in any way. What matters is what *we* do. For example, I have a friend in Dallas who, over the last twenty years, has consistently lost money in real estate. This takes a certain talent because, until a few years ago, real estate in Dallas was only going up.

So what goes on around us is irrelevant. It is what we do that matters. With that understanding, we begin to observe the process by which a spirit arises in us and is articulated as our life experience. The process of observing that spirit both within us and in everything around us is the focus of the next phase of practice called shaktopaya.

Shaktopaya

The sun is reflected both in the salty waves of the sea and in the clear surface of a mountain lake. Seeing things with the physical eyes is not enough. You must experience the inner significance of the thing seen.

— NITYANANDA

Introduction

The effect of anavopaya is the stilling of our minds. We engage our lives in the world around us with a spirit of lightness, ease, and grace. This is not just a matter of turning down the radio between our ears or learning exercises to relax our bodies. It is a qualitative change in the way we engage in our experience.

What defines it as anavopaya in particular is that our perception of that experience is still primarily dualistic. We think of everything in terms of "I" and "something other," a subject and an object. So the sense of well-being we experience is in terms of how we perceive the relationship between that "I" and "other."

But if reality is only one thing, then even this is still a form of ignorance. We may get along a lot better in the world, which is a wonderful thing, but we have still not gone beyond the fundamental confusion that got us into the soup in the first place. Shaktopaya, the strategy involving awareness of the energy of Life Itself, lifts us out of this level of confusion.

The basic elements of our practice — finding a real teacher and beginning to work with him or her, mastering technique, and extending ourselves to serve whatever situation we find ourselves in — are really only the starting points of our inner work. Even to say that our work is essentially about releasing tensions and allowing our creative energy to flow is a statement with many layers to it.

When we start out, we are mostly aware of the work involved in releasing tensions. We are learning to drop our habits of reaction and defensiveness in favor of opening our hearts and remaining open even in the face of tremendous pressure and pain. Different parts of our conditioning start to fall away, and we find that things we thought were intrinsic parts of our personalities are not. Most of all we begin to be aware of the presence of something deeper at work in and around us.

As that happens, we recognize the limitations of effort, struggle, and control. Our attention begins to shift from the aspect of our work that involves effort, and we become increasingly aware of the dynamic nature of the Presence we experience when we sit in meditation. When we pay attention to it, we notice it more and more as the underlying quality of our lives and of the different environments in which we move.

We open ourselves deeply to the pulsation of this energy of Life Itself. This pulsation the Trika masters called spanda. We start to experience everything as an expression of spanda and its creative flow. The circumstances in which we find ourselves may not have changed in the least, but our perception of them makes them something entirely different to us from what they were.

In the same way, we continue with all the basic elements of our practice, doing each day just what we did from the first. Yet we discover that these things, too, we see with a difference. The Trika thinkers summed up the essence of this difference in their increasingly refined discussions of spanda and the three foundational elements of our practice: our relationship with the teacher, meditation, and the ways in which we extend our energy. They said that, increasingly, we experience these things as energy. In the following chapters we will talk about what this means.

The basic insight the Trika masters came to was that there is a unity underneath all the diversity. The basis of that unity is the energy. Even while a person remains aware of the differences between things he or she can also be deeply aware that they are not just *parts* of one thing, but one thing itself — the energy. So they called the awareness that emerges in this phase of practice the awareness of unity-in-diversity. We see things as multiple and as one, both at the same time. This is the awareness of the energy: shaktopaya.

The Strategy of the Energy

SPANDA: THE ENERGY OF LIFE ITSELF

Feel the life force flowing from you and drawing into you from the atmosphere: from the rain, from the sky, from the air around you and the sky above you, and the stars and the moon and the sun, and everything that exists that represents energy.

— RUDI

A Dynamic Stillness

As we learn to quiet our minds, we become increasingly aware of the energy of Life Itself that permeates all our experience. Indeed, the heart of our inner work involves coming to know and immerse ourselves in that energy. If this is true for us, it was no less true for the ancient masters of Trika Yoga. Their own spiritual practice was the laboratory in which they discovered and explored this infinite energy, called spanda.

When the early Trika masters looked for ways to talk about their experience of spanda, they pointed to different encounters with the world around them to say what it was like. Their most basic insight was that the infinite is not merely energy, but conscious energy. This is the foundation of all reality as we know it.

111

It is, they went on to say, a pure awareness that is utterly still. At the same time, this conscious energy is dynamic. This is because Life is not only stillness but also motion and vitality. So right from the start they were asserting a paradox about the Absolute, saying that it is both a stillness and a dynamic vitality. God, they said, is a dynamic stillness.

If this seems difficult to grasp, take as an analogy the way particle physics has demonstrated that matter and energy are one and the same. All matter, if observed submicroscopically, consists of energy. A particle, if observed in one way, appears to be matter, a kind of stillness. From another perspective, it is pure energy and behaves as a wave. Moreover, both things are always true of it.

Likewise, think of your own experience in which there is always a part of you that is still and a part that is in motion. At any given time, one aspect or the other predominates. There is more than just a connection between what is still and what is dynamic; on a larger scale, they become two aspects of the same thing.

If this is true in our own limited experience, it is no less true at the level of the highest reality, where pure awareness and dynamic, creative energy are completely interpenetrated. They are a single reality. That is why the iconography of Shaivism depicts the Absolute as the intimate embrace of two lovers, Shiva and Shakti. It is a way of representing the nature of this field of energy and giving us an idea of the relationship between them. It shows them not as two things but one. This is a visual image of dynamic stillness.

In the tradition of our practice, the aspect of pure awareness is called Shiva. In the iconography, this is represented as masculine and passive. The dynamic aspect is called Shakti, or energy. It is also called spanda. Shakti is shown as feminine and active. Shiva, being essentially passive, is shown with one form; Shakti, being active, is often shown with many. Everything that has to do with the Absolute extending and expressing itself as manifest reality is Shakti, or spanda.

When we talk about this whole event we talk about it as two things: There is consciousness and there is energy; there is passive awareness and vitality; there is stillness and manifestation. Ultimately, however, both are one and the same.

"Shakti" and "spanda" are also two different words for the same thing. The difference is that Shakti is a kind of personification, represented visually as a goddess, which gives a gender and identity to this energy. Spanda, on the other hand, is a technical term that refers to the dynamic aspect of the highest level of consciousness.

The term "spanda" means a throb or vibration. It is the creative pulsation of Life Itself. Its root meaning refers to something "having a slight movement." This is not movement as we usually think of it, however. Since the Absolute is also infinite stillness, this pulsation is more the throbbing of Life's dynamism, which appears as if moving. It is not actual physical motion but the infinite pulsation of the divine creative energy.

Spanda is also described as a kind of potency, or potentiality, that is present everywhere and always. Sometimes it is described as a pregnancy. It refers to the inherent capacity of Life Itself for growth and creative Self-expression. It is a vital awareness that has not yet articulated itself in, or as, time and space but is poised on the edge of doing so. We can also say it is a choiceless awareness, in the sense that it has not yet taken on — or chosen — a specific articulation.

This means that, at this level of pure potentiality, there is neither past nor future, but only present. What is the quality of this present? Again, it is a dynamic stillness. It is the moment *between* events, the point right before something happens. It is the pregnant stillness out of which anything and everything can come.

For example, when a musician sits down at the piano and raises his or her hands to strike the keys for the first time, that moment's pause is pregnant with possibility. At the same time, it is utterly still. It has the quality of being beyond time and space, in a present that is infinite.

This moment of perfect poise is the essential condition of the unity of Shiva and Shakti. There is no actual movement, but the power of infinite vitality is completely there. It is that pure awareness which is the foundation of every creative expression.

The Expression of Spanda

So how does this pure potential turn into the reality that we encounter every day? Think of some occasion when you were walking down the street feeling terrific. Something inside you suddenly gives a subtle throb, and maybe you take a little skip-step. Maybe you start to whistle or sing. In other words, you do something to express yourself for no reason except that you feel so good you cannot help it.

With the divine it is essentially the same. As Shakti, God expresses itself because of the vitality — we could even say the exuberance — of God's own nature. After all, if you were infinite, you would be not only infinitely aware, you would also be infinitely free and creative, and infinitely joyful. The whole universe, including us, is an expression of such a throb of exuberance. It is the rapture of the divine manifesting as a spontaneous, purposeless expression of sheer joy. We may have little or no awareness of this, but it is no less true.

Spanda is like an infinite heartbeat. It is a subtle agitation in an infinite medium in which no real distinctions of time and place are possible. Its throb is equidistant throughout an infinite energy field; it is equally powerful and equally present throughout the entire medium.

This infinite field of energy cannot have a single center. If it did, it would no longer be infinite. So, in a sense, this makes every point in this infinity the source of the creative throb of spanda. Every point is its center, and every point has equal power. The result is a subtle, seething, simmering situation — a pulsating, dynamic event.

All these simultaneous pulsations interact with each other, and their interaction gives rise to multiple vibrations. A medium in which a pulsation arises from infinite centers becomes something like boiling water. The interaction of one vibration with another gives rise to many frequencies. The process is one in which everything is expanding and contracting equally from every single point, generating the appearance of waves. The multiple vibrations generated by the vitality of spanda are like that.

In a very real way the whole world is a vital ocean of conscious energy, of potentiality. If we go to the edge of the ocean, we see waves rising and falling. However, if we look down on the water from a high place, what we might see are really pulses of energy moving through an entirely passive, fluid medium. Even when we see waves coming in and going out, the water is not actually traveling horizontally. The movement of the water molecules is really up and down. It is just a pulse of energy. Moreover, even though the pulse of energy and the water itself are not the same thing, they are also not separate.

In the ocean a multitude of major, minor, and still finer currents all interact with each other. At the same time each of these currents is only water moving at one rate of speed relative to the water on either side of it. It is not different water even if it seems set apart by the movement.

Some areas move faster, while others move more slowly, so that there seem to be different densities of water within the medium. These different densities also have different vibrations. The point is that currents within currents within currents are constantly manifesting in this medium, which is nothing but consciousness.

This is not like dropping a rock in a pond and having the ripples radiate outward. Rather it is like dropping an infinite number of rocks in a pond and watching the waves interact with each other. Each interaction creates many smaller centers of interaction, and so on and so forth. The universe is something like this, except that there is no external force that generates this dynamic pulsation. It generates itself from all points within itself.

The word resonance gives us a proper flavor for what happens. Certain frequencies of energy resonate with each other and come together in ways that are greater than the sum of the parts. Thus we have a field of infinite conscious energy, bulging with potential at every point. These bulges, bumping into each other from every potential point within the medium, lead to the appearance of what we call our reality.

As this energy becomes further articulated, it takes on the appearance of what we talk about as light. Light, slowed down to six hundred and fifty miles an hour, becomes sound, although it is still energy. Slowed down even further, it becomes matter. In this sense, we can think of sound as substance, and matter as form. So the dynamic stillness of this infinite presence expresses itself as the appearance of all substance and form. As it does so, it takes on the appearance of many apparently separate lives, like our own.

Expansion, Contraction, and Stillpoints

A fundamental organizing principle underlies this whole process: Any pulsation is really an alternation between expansion and contraction. As the energy of Life articulates and expresses itself, there is an expansion. Whatever comes forth in this expansion is sustained for a while in time and space, and has a function. Then it contracts and dissolves back into its original medium.

Although individual forms come and go, the one constant is this expansion and contraction of the energy. On each and every level of life this organizing principle, which the ancient texts refer to as the dual aspect of spanda, acts as a consistent pattern. This is the changeless principle underlying all change.

This organizing pattern also has an evolutionary component because it has the creative freedom to change and evolve — to respond to changes of pressure, frequency, and vibration in the immediate environment. This means that we have a perpetually dynamic event existing in, and operating on, multiple dimensions.

Are extension and absorption always happening simultaneously? This is a tricky question. In one sense they are. Still, from our perspective as individuals, they don't happen at the same time. For example, in a wave coming onto the beach, extension and retraction are happening at the same time. A new wave comes in even as the old wave is being pulled back. There is the continuous appearance of both things happening at the same time. Nevertheless, we notice one aspect more than another at any given moment, depending on where we focus our attention.

The pulsation of Life extends and contracts itself within parameters called stillpoints, or *bindus*. Any pulsation naturally extends itself to a certain point, pauses, and then recedes, something like the ocean tides. Any manifestation in time and space, regardless of how subtle or gross, has such parameters. This is a constant cycle. The stillpoints that come about when something is either fully extended or has fully receded — the pauses before the process reverses and takes another direction — are inherent in every dynamic situation. Without stillpoints, a vibratory field cannot occur.

In our own experience, for example, we encounter these stillpoints in our own breathing, at the end of an inhalation just before we exhale and at the end of an exhalation just before we inhale. In those pauses, if we pay attention, we encounter the essence of the dynamic stillness of spanda. If we listen, the quality of those moments tells us everything about the nature of God.

The practical reason for this discussion is understanding that all experience is inseparable from the essential flow and pulsation of spanda. The universal creative power does not have boundaries but parameters. These parameters are operational, and we experience them. This is what allows us to become aware of the fundamental rhythm of any experience and also of the rhythm of our lives. When we train ourselves to become aware of this pulsation of Life Itself, we discover that these stillpoints permeate our lives. Ultimately we recognize that everything is the stillpoint.

The Interchange of Infinite Energy

Spanda underlies the manifestation of everything. This includes wars, famines, and pestilence just as much as it includes families, picnics, fine moments, happy lives, and acts of courage and self-sacrifice. Within the whole, many different scenes play themselves out. The point is that spanda manifests in every possible form and that all experiences, without exception, are implicit in the subtle potency that is the vitality of consciousness.

Consciousness, in its Shakti aspect, is constantly and even violently in such motion. If we look at the universe, we see — even though its vast spaces make it seem highly impersonal — that our physical universe is always in motion. We may not recognize it to the same degree within our bodies, but it is going on there, too. We experience, to some extent, the motion going on in the field of our individual experience, but because our senses limit our perceptions, it is easy for us to ignore or tune it out. Nevertheless, on every level, there is always this constant dynamic.

On every level we are nothing but networks of energy. Having experienced themselves in this way through their spiritual practice, the Trika philosophers went on to understand the world in the same way, as lines of force arising from the fundamental field of energy. Moreover, even though these lines of force come out of this field they are not distinct from it. The universe, these teachers said, is a network of such energies.

Ultimately, we want to understand that our own creative energy, along with the network of energies as a whole, is nothing but the creative energy of the divine. If we can absorb that understanding, we see that the creative energy manifesting itself through everyone in the whole world is one and the same. Then instead of being aware of *things* interacting, we see everything as the interchange of infinite, conscious energy.

The mind, of course, has difficulty with the idea of infinite energy. Think of it this way, though. Have you ever had a moment of profound and utter joy? Did it end? You might say, "Well, it ended about fifteen minutes ago." Maybe. But maybe it was more the case that something else happened to shift your attention away from that experience of joy. This is different from saying that the experience itself ended. It did not end and, in reality, never does. The amazing thing about it is that it actually goes on forever.

When we cultivate our awareness of this reality, we discover it has no boundaries. This is not an understanding we can conceptualize. It is not possible to grasp or envision something that goes beyond conception and envisioning. Indeed the very act of grasping denies us the understanding we want. This is an understanding to which we can only open ourselves. This opening we call surrender.

Surrender, in this case, means that we have to quiet our minds and let this understanding flow from within us. Then there is no grasping but only a releasing. We release our need to conceptualize, and slowly it dawns on us what this infinity, which is simple and subtle, is all about.

One of the extraordinary things we come to recognize is that the reality we think we know so well does not operate as we usually think it does. For that matter, it is nothing like what we imagine it to be. For example, it is difficult for us to get, in terms of our daily experience, that there is really no such thing as "matter." What we think of as matter exists for a moment, and then dissipates. Even when it exists, it is ninety or ninety-eight percent space. In the big picture, we ourselves exist within a medium in which we coalesce for only a short period of time and then disperse.

No form is truly solid. What we take to be forms are more like the aurora borealis, shimmering curtains of light high up in the northern skies. The energy of Life Itself happens like this at every point in time and space. From the perspective of the infinite, everything has form and loses it in such a way that both the having and the losing occur simultaneously. This description is one hundred and eighty degrees different from the understanding on which we base how we ordinarily think and do things.

Although some people are born who have never lost their awareness of this, for most of us it is a case of having to suspend the rational process and allow what lies behind our thoughts and minds to flow into our awareness. This awareness is particularly difficult to conceive of when we are locked into the perspective of our individual separateness. As long as we are defending our individuation, how can we sense our-selves as connected to the whole and intuit the fundamental ground from which we arise? Even when we sense a deeper reality, our awareness of it is clouded over almost as quickly.

To give you an analogy, suppose you are sitting quietly at home, feeling focused and centered. Suddenly the dog comes along, wags its tail, and starts to knock a cup off the table. You dive for it. In doing so, you lose some of your sense of being centered. It is not that your center disappears, but your attention and concentration get distracted by the degree to which you shift your focus outside of yourself during that moment of action.

This is referred to in the texts as the obscuring of the highest state. This tendency toward action can cloud our experience of that expansive state for eons. We lock our atten-tion on actions and their outcomes, whether in the form of careers, missions, or any number of other things. The end result is that we lose contact with the subtle, expansive state. This is why the Trika thinkers looked for the means to act without their awareness ever being obscured, to move in the world without ever experiencing any alienation from their innate, universal condition. They wanted to find ways to sus-tain the awareness that even though everything has an appear-ance of separateness, there is also a unity to our existence that makes the fullness of Life Itself available to every person. The unity in all of this, from the simplest to the most complex manifestation of Life, is the principle of Spanda.

Everything is nothing but the energy of Life Itself. Everything we see and feel, everything we think we know, and even everything we think, is nothing but a shadow, a reflection of the presence that is real, that is here and now, and that in no way is as it appears. We can see it clearly not with our physical eyes but when we quiet our minds. Then, out of the corners of our eyes, we see the real behind the shadow.

I said that in the course of expressing itself as manifest reality, the true nature of the absolute is concealed. What does this mean? It means that the one, interacting with itself, takes on the appearance of the many and covers over its real nature, as though putting on veils. It is actually one of the characteristics of the divine to conceal its real nature. Likewise, it is also one of its characteristics to reveal that same nature. The latter expresses itself as our inner longing to know the deeper aspect of who we are.

The Tattvas

Part of the challenge the early Trika masters faced was to explain the actual process by which the one becomes many. In a general way, they talked about this as the spanda principle of pulsation. Through their own inner work, however, they also refined this discussion into many subtle phases.

The issue was this: How does the conscious energy of the divine, which experiences everything as its own Self, become transformed into an awareness of "I," and "this" or "that" — an awareness of multiplicity in which there is a subject and an object? How does this further articulate itself as the material universe and, within that, as human beings?

In exploring the dynamic process by which the world comes into manifestation, these masters broke it down into thirty-six phases that range from absolutely pure, dynamic consciousness, to the elements that compose the material world. They developed this analysis by examining their own consciousness and the power underlying their minds, emotions, and physical experiences, and by understanding this power as the dynamic underlying all evolutionary processes.

This is an important point. These were people committed to practice and to a lived-through experience. They did not come up with this discussion as a matter of abstract speculation. Rather this was a language they developed to describe what they had discovered in the course of their practice. From that they developed techniques and commentaries to transmit these experiences and insights to their students. These insights are equally meaningful to our own inner work because what these teachers were getting at was that things are not as they appear to be. They were trying to come up with ways to show precisely how this is so.

Using themselves as laboratories, they anticipated in extraordinary ways some of the observations of modern physics regarding the formation of the universe, in which energy interacts with itself to form increasingly dense clusters of matter and, ultimately, galaxies and solar systems in all their details. The element that sets the Trika masters apart is their assertion that the energy out of which all reality emerges is conscious. There is, therefore, nothing that does not participate in the essential quality of awareness.

They called the actual phases of this process *tattvas*. "Tattva" means a principle; in this case a principle of manifestation. It refers to the way in which the universe unfolds. It also means the essence, the real condition or state of something, the "thatness" or "suchness" of a thing or event.

The first people to write on this subject and to postulate the presence of these principles were part of a school of thought called Samkhya. They asserted the existence of twenty-five tattvas, or phases of unfoldment. The Trika thinkers expanded these to thirty-six. So although they did not originate the discussion of tattvas, they greatly refined it.

This discussion becomes more immediately pertinent to our own experience of our lives in terms of how the Self undergoes a series of phases until it takes on a limited and fragmented perception of itself as an individuated self. This happens because of what are known as the tattvas of individual experience and particularly because of what is called *maya tattva*, or *maya*. The Sanskrit root *ma* means "to measure out," and maya tattva is the process by which experience becomes measurable, finite, and separate.

In this process, all the qualities of the infinite creative pulsation of Life Itself crystallize into more limited forms. It is something like starting out with a very loose garment that can hold everything in the world, and then washing and putting it in the dryer, and having it shrink down very small. All its original elements are still there, but in a shrunken form. If it still fits, it does so only in the narrowest sense. Then we get used to wearing a size contracted instead of a size infinite, and forget how big the thing really is.

Maya gives rise to the fundamental confusion over the Self. It leads to our general belief that we consist of bodies, minds, emotions, and so on. We operate with a highly constricted idea of what constitutes *us*, in which infinite "Self" becomes individualized "self." So in our daily lives the infinite Self enters our experience as the ego, the empirical "me." In addition, since we think of our bodies as part of our basic reality, we buy into the idea that we are actually distinct from the reality around us.

For example, we assume that when our bodies die, so do we. We don't see that if we are fundamentally nothing but conscious energy, then even though our form dissolves back into a larger field of energy, nothing really dies. What is alive about us is always alive.

Maya brings about a contracted experience of ourselves in five specific ways known as the five *kanchukas*: First, the infinite power of the creative energy of Life Itself is reduced to individual actions. Since we identify with our bodies, we imagine we are bounded by our capacity for limited activity. Then we start judging these actions. We decide that some of them are good and others bad. These leave their impressions on us in the form of tensions.

Second, the omniscience of the infinite becomes a limited knowledge of a fragmented reality. This is the finite understanding with which we are accustomed to dealing with the world. It is based on our having the perception of subjects and objects because knowledge is always "about" something that we take to be "other." The paradox is that both the subject and the objects that we perceive are nothing but contractions in infinite consciousness. So ultimately all subjects and objects are the same as Shiva: one thing.

In this way we get caught up in particulars and believe them to be true elements in our experience. We buy into the apparent reality of the distinctions between things without seeing that all the particulars are the myriad expressions of that one, deeper reality. This way of seeing things is the territory of the mind, which is encumbered by these perceptions of difference and by all the structures that seem integral to reality. This is why Rudi always referred to the mind as the slayer of the soul.

Third, the sense of joy and total well-being that character-izes the energy of Life Itself contracts into distinct longings and desires for specific things. Then instead of our happiness being an innate quality of our being, we look for it in things outside ourselves. This is not so surprising once we lose our feeling of our own highest reality. We scatter our energy in pursuit of people, places, and things, trying to satisfy our desires and fulfill our appetites.

What we don't realize is that in the process we become subject to our desires and perpetually agitated by them. Instead of really being able to enjoy them, they begin to enjoy *us*. That is, they eat us alive. We become bound into our efforts to satisfy them in an unending round of limited pleasures.

Fourth, the eternity of the infinite is reduced, or mea-sured out, into limitations with regard to time. Once we are talking about things that arise, last for a while, and then dis-solve, we are talking about past, present, and future. At the level of the absolute, no time exists. In the infinite there is nothing but an infinite present. On our own level of individ-ual experience, however, we are frequently ruled by our experience of time, trapped by our sense of the past, appre-hensive about our sense of the future, and unable to feel at ease in the present. Moreover, it doesn't occur to us that time as we know it has nothing to do with the experience of the highest state of awareness.

Finally, once we see ourselves as distinct from everything else, and everything else as separate events all operating in time, it follows that we perceive ourselves to be acting *upon* the people, places, and things around us. Likewise, we experi-ence them as acting upon each other and upon us. Out of the infinite freedom of the creative energy, then, there arises the experience of cause and effect operating in space.

These are the five ways in which we are crystallized expressions of the creative energy of Life Itself. Together, they are like an illusory overlay, masking authentic life. They lead us to identify with the effects of particular forms of experience, instead of with pure experience itself. Their net effect is to direct our attention increasingly outside of ourselves.

Our spiritual work is the process by which we become more and more deeply aware of the energy at the core of every overlay until we experience that energy as the essence of all things, including ourselves. At first we are aware of distinctions. This is the awareness of anavopaya. Then we come to see a basic unity between all aspects of reality, even as some sense of distinction persists. This is the awareness of shaktopaya. Finally we experience *all* of reality as an expression of the Self. This is the awareness of shambhavopaya. Each phase of awareness is a way of perceiving and experiencing the creative energy of Life Itself.

Through our contact with a teacher, through our practice, and as we learn to extend our energy, we become more and more aware of the things I have talked about in connection with spanda. We experience the pulsation and its stillpoints, the process of manifestation through the tattvas, and the ways in which we ourselves are contracted expressions of the fundamental energy of Life. Thus as we learn to take our attention inside and stabilize it there, the insights of the masters of Trika Yoga become our own.

THE GURU

These teachings exist as an energy. And the energy, this abstract quantity, is what we are really after. People always think they can gain learning, knowledge, and wisdom by taking a teaching in words. Words only represent the shell, or the crust, of knowledge.

— RUDI

From Personality to Energy

As beginning students we seek contact with the teacher. We look for opportunities to approach him or her as instructor, counselor, and even friend. At this level of interaction, we seek information, advice, and a sense of connection. In the process we get caught up in different ways of trying to figure out how to relate to this other individual. We look at the reality of surrender that we meet in the teacher, and confront our own resistance to growing. So as beginning students part of our experience of the teacher is one of struggle and effort.

The other part, if we are with an authentic teacher, is the experience of a flow and of contact with a deeper awareness to which we have access through our interaction with him or her. This is because the function of a teacher is, first of all, to arouse our awareness of that energy flow in ways we don't yet know how to do for ourselves. He or she trains us in a set of skills and puts us in touch with the fundamental vitality that is our essence. As rookies and beginners it doesn't matter much that we don't know how to generate it ourselves all that well. Basically, in this phase the teacher does most of the work for us anyway, and what we experience is a function of the work we do directly with him or her.

Our contact with the teacher gives us the occasion to attune ourselves to that resonance in action. We establish a level of rapport with it and then learn to sustain and build upon it. This means that as beginning students, when we sit in meditation with a teacher, it does not exactly matter whether we are doing everything the way we are supposed to or not. Either way, the refinement process is taking place.

As we sit together, it doesn't matter whether we feel we are taking in energy, or awakening or arousing it from within ourselves. What does matter is that we are not in our heads but opening deeply within ourselves and feeling the flow of energy there. On some days we will think it is moving from inside us outward; on others we will think it is entering us from outside. After a while we understand that it is both. *It* is really breathing *us*, and we are an extension of *it*, not vice versa.

Real contact or connection with a guru enables us to feel so deeply secure and calm that we can begin to turn within and observe the workings of our inner universe without the doubts, fears, and tensions that ordinarily draw our minds back into the realm of dualistic awareness. At the same time, our contact with the teacher trains us to steady ourselves in the awareness of the energy so that this awareness is more continuously in the foreground, regardless of whatever particular situation we find ourselves in. For this to happen, however, a shift in our perception of the teacher must come about, a shift related to two aspects of the teacher.

On one level we are engaging with another individual. He or she is a personality to be dealt with and talked to, a person who performs actions that have an effect on the world, a person viewed by some with respect and admiration and rejected by others with disgust. In other words, a human being viewed by other people as ordinary, the same or less then they themselves.

At this level we are subject to our likes and dislikes, our judgments and values, and our feelings about that other personality. All these things enter into our perceptions of the teacher. Moreover, insofar as we *are* dealing with another human being, we will probably continue to notice these things.

It is also altogether likely at this stage of our work with the teacher that every kind of impurity, limitation, obstacle, and misunderstanding within us is going to surface. Either we are going to absorb it all as energy and go beyond the tension, or we are going to allow it to crystallize and look for some place to dump it all — usually on the teacher. At that point it becomes the limit of our ability to grow.

Some people do well for a while. They make a little progress and become proud of themselves. Then they get stuck there and say, "Oh, this whole process of serving a teacher is really full of it." They recoil and cut the connection, in which case their ideas about duality and the basic difficulty out of which they emerged in the first place snaps back on them faster than you can snap your fingers, and more powerfully than ever before.

So one of the most powerful ways our resistance to releasing tensions expresses itself can be in our reaction to the teacher, one of whose functions is to mirror back to us our own tensions. What we bring to the interaction is what we get back. This means there will be all kinds of times when the rapport is strained over issues of personality, times when we have to be careful and full of surrender in order to be sure our own program is not getting in the way.

Yet the real issue is never one of liking or not liking the teacher. As Rudi pointed out, you can meet a saint you don't like and still benefit by being in that presence. Our job is to draw the energy into ourselves as nourishment. It is for us to go beyond all the blocks of personality in order to harmonize the relationship. At the same time, it is up to the teacher to help us remove the obstacles to the flow when we make a sincere effort to do so.

The most important thing is to find within the teacher what it is we wish to learn, and to draw this energy into ourselves. Our job is to see beyond the form, transcend the personality and eccentricities, and go beyond even the things we dislike. In so doing, we go beyond our own personalities and limitations. When we can see beyond the form of the physical teacher, we become aware of the power that functions as and through the guru. Then it becomes our work to still our minds in the flow of that energy.

The human aspect of the guru, or what Nityananda called the secondary teacher, acts like a doorway. We pass through it to the level of consciousness that Nityananda called the primary guru. He said that the secondary guru leads us to the well, while the primary guru drinks from it. When this happens, we enter our work as advanced students, in which we encounter the teacher not primarily as a personality but as an extraordinary field of spiritual energy. From this field we draw deep nourishment and grow in spiritual maturity.

By taking our attention inside and becoming aware of the nature of this energy field, we obtain a dramatically changed awareness of ourselves. Follow the logic. Suppose you and I are sitting together, looking at each other. You are aware of strong experience points within yourself. Then you begin to be aware of something that connects the two of us. You feel a subtle expansion take place into a field of connection. In that expansion of the energy you may experience a subtle tremor as your attention shifts from your awareness of yourself as a separate individual with a whole range of thoughts, feelings, wants, and needs, to an awareness of participating in a broader field of energy that encompasses other centers of awareness — namely, both of us.

This then expands to become an awareness of the field itself and of its nature, which is, in a way, independent of all this individuality. Then we go beyond even the experience of that dynamic to become aware of the pure, subtle ground from which it emerges, only to realize that we ourselves are nothing other than that ourselves.

In a simple experience like this we go through a condensed version of what it is like to transcend personality. The point is that when we can go beyond the individual limitations of the teacher, we can also go beyond our own. Then we meet in the place where limitations have no more meaning than currents passing through the water.

Shaktipat

According to the *Shiva Sutras*, an eighth century foundation text of Kashmir Shaivism, "The guru is the means." When I first read this, I recalled my initial experience of Rudi. I imagined him to be something like a dimensional warp, a hole in the universe of time and space. I understood that if I were going to find God and become established in that truth, I would have to go through Rudi. I don't mean that he was going to take me out and introduce me to it, but that where I wanted to go was literally through him.

This might seem, at first, to be a somewhat difficult proposition. Rudi was wide, so it was not easy to get around him; he was thick, which meant one was not going to get through him in any ordinary sense of the word; and he was strong, which made me think he might not like it if someone were to push into him. So I understood that going through him didn't mean I was going to crawl inside him in any way.

Rather it meant I would become so attuned to him that the energy *he* was would be present for me. I would connect to and be transformed by it totally, and therefore be free. That this happened was for one reason: because I trusted him totally. Through this I learned about trusting in the energy of Life Itself. This was how I came to understand the idea that the guru is the means.

This relationship to the energy that we encounter in the guru takes on an explicit form in the practice of Trika Yoga through what is known as *shaktipat*. What defines a real teacher more than anything else, and what sets the Kashmir Shaivite tradition apart from others, is the practice and experience of shaktipat. This means "the descent of the energy," or "the transmission of the teaching." It is also referred to as divine grace.

Shaktipat has its roots in an ancient Indian tradition that continues to permeate Indian culture, namely the tradition of *darshan*. Darshan means "seeing," and refers to the practice of seeing the image of the deity and hoping that the deity will see you back. This approach is one way of talking about looking into the face of God, and recognizing that what we find in that experience is intimate and ultimate at the same time. This understanding of the mechanism by which blessings are bestowed and teaching transmitted exists in India everywhere from the most unsophisticated and commercialized forms of worship to the most refined. For example, the whole point of going to a temple is to look upon the figure of the deity in a spirit of deep devotion. This is felt to be of great benefit in and of itself. It is even more beneficial to be seen, oneself, through the eyes of the deity.

In the Trika Yoga system an important part of the interactive ritual between student and teacher consists of eye contact with the teacher who, it is said, installs him- or herself in the student. That is, he or she transmits a creative energy and force to the student. In the context of the earliest and most radical of the ascetic practitioners, this probably took place spontaneously. As this happened, and as people recognized it to be a mechanism of transmission, slowly it became structured into rituals. By the eleventh century the Trika master Abhinava-gupta describes a highly ritualized form of it as well as a more spontaneous form.

This eyes-open event, called both *bhairava mudra* and *krama mudra*, is the most refined aspect of Tantric ritual. Traditionally, people without the openness or understanding necessary for that glance to penetrate their awareness were trained in many preliminary techniques to prepare them for it. For example, they were given many mantras to recite to bring them to the point of openness where that transmission could take place.

The point of all contact with the teacher, and what is transmitted, is what is known as the vital breath. The teacher may look into the eyes of the student, or may apply what is referred to as the hand of Shiva, or the touch. The metaphor in each case is that first there are two. Because of the transmission of the energy, the vital breath, these two become one. A kind of fusion happens, which is the entry-point by which a person begins to recognize the unity of all things. Awakened by grace, we penetrate the mystery and recognize ourselves to be nothing but the Self, or Shiva.

Shaktipat itself can also happen, the texts say, on three levels: weak, medium, and strong. In the case of weak shaktipat, it is like having a broken mechanism that gets fixed. In the medium, a stuck mechanism gets released and energized. In the strong, the mechanism itself is destroyed; that is, all structure and pattern dissolve into a greater whole. Along with the destruction of the mechanism comes the end of desire, ambition, want, and need. There is the end of getting or giving, or any such ideas. So, in a sense, weak shaktipat makes a person happy, medium shaktipat makes a person able, and strong shaktipat makes a person free.

It is not that shaktipat exists for some and not for others; it exists for everybody. This is because the circumstances of every person's life are fundamentally the same. It is the entanglement in our desires and the feedback of our worldly lives that causes us to remain stuck in the lowest level of feedback which denies us the recognition of that potency. Some people continue to pursue that feedback until they die, while others, for some reason, wake up and smell the coffee.

What takes us beyond being caught up in the narrowest kinds of feedback can only be spoken of as grace, just as what enters our lives through shaktipat and our connection with the teacher is also the experience of grace. This refers to the quality that is the essence of our experience when we live from within. Each person attracts around him- or herself a life experience based upon the vibration that he or she carries internally.

We are each of us like a tuning fork. You can feel this yourself. All you have to do is be quiet for a little bit and you will feel the multiplicity of vibrations that are within you. From the unstructured creative energy of life which is both material and non-material, we attract and organize around ourselves a life experience. Grace is that life experience that arises from within and around us when we are attuned to the simplest, finest vibration available within us. That experience we call grace because it has a sweetness, freshness, and vitality to it that allow us to be joyful in the face of whatever happens.

Our experience of shaktipat gives us the direct experience of this. It brings about a quantum leap in our awareness that puts us in contact with the innate freedom and spontaneous creative power eternally and everywhere present as the source of all. It awakens the deepest potentiality within us, allowing the energy to begin its extraordinary unfoldment within us.

In the process the transmission of the energy is understood to sever the bonds of the student to the life he or she had known. It releases all commitments, obligations, and tensions of every kind. In India, for example, it releases a person from the bonds of caste. In our case, shaktipat is the creative energy that burns away our illusions and misunderstandings, our habits of mind, and our bondage to convention. It is this descent of grace that begins to loosen up all the tensions and other mechanisms we have developed to compensate for the pain in our lives. It is also what allows us to move toward the restoration of our own free and interdependent condition. I say "interdependent" because when we understand our own nature more deeply, we recognize how profoundly connected we all really are.

Shaktipat awakens us to the infinite power that is the support and the source of our individuated existence. It is that experience of release that allows us to recognize a deeper conscious power functioning from within us, whose capacity in every way infinitely exceeds our own. Ideally such an experience puts an end to selfishness and individual self-absorption, pride and arrogance, egotism and ambition, and every desire. Through this contact, tension and stuckness dissolve and we realize our highest condition.

As this unfoldment continues, our entire structure is refined and purified. When iron is subjected to fire, it is freed of its gross crystallization and impurities as it reorganizes into the finer, stronger form of steel. We also, by passing through the forge of the guru, become refined by the inner fire of the energy.

This happens in our lives through our interaction with the teacher to the degree that we most deeply want it to. This is easy to say, of course, but think about it. To the degree that we are committed to going beyond every limitation and finite understanding of ourselves, our experience of shaktipat will release us. So it has an impact on us directly according to our longing for it to do so.

Another way of saying this is that it is a function of our capacity to surrender — to open ourselves profoundly. This means that it happens to a willing student. Indeed, a willing student is all it takes. It doesn't particularly take a willing teacher. For that matter, the less will present in the teacher, the better for the situation, because it is from the state of surrender in the teacher that the transmission of the experience of the infinite Self takes place, and not from will. Nevertheless, the teacher is the unifying principle underlying every experience of shaktipat.

This experience has nothing to do with words. Even though the teacher may instruct us in the texts of the tradition and should, in fact, have an intuitive grasp of their contents, the real teaching occurs as the energy of the student rises to meet the energy descending from the teacher. There is no substitute for this communion. This is why in all the highest, most refined manifestations of spiritual teaching in Asia, the teacher is of fundamental importance. If we look at Jesus as a teacher, we see this is also true in Christianity.

Meditation is what we do every day to keep this communion going, although meditation does not make it happen in the first place. Rather our inner wish and our participation in the broader energy field bring it about. Nor is there any getting around the work we must do to draw on what we receive, in order to internalize, digest, and grow from it. In this work we discover ever more deeply that what we are exploring is love itself, just as the center in which we establish ourselves is that love. Whatever shape, color, form, or texture it may assume, this is the essence of our work with the teacher.

The Teacher as a Rhythm

The nature of the whole universe, as we have seen in the discussion of spanda, is vibration. This is sometimes referred to as the dance of Shiva. Neither our own consciousness or anything else exists outside of this vibration. As we refine our practice, we realize that our participation in the teaching is actually the process of cultivating our awareness not of the teacher as an individual, but of the rhythm of the teacher and the rhythm of the teaching. We train ourselves, through our commitment and concentration, to carry our awareness of that rhythm through our day. It is our experience of it that matters, as well as our ability to reconnect to it over and over again regardless of where we are.

Nor does it have to take long. For example, it takes me only seconds to connect to that rhythm that was Rudi's specific frequency. Every individual teacher has such a rhythm. On an obvious level, for example, Rudi talked with a specific cadence. When he sat down to teach class, there was a rhythm to that, too. But the rhythm I am talking about is the underlying field of the teaching in which we are attempting to participate. The rhythm represents the basic frequency on which the teaching is being transmitted. That living rhythm we encounter is what teaches us, and not the finite individual. The more we become aware of and attuned to it, the more quickly we recognize it not only in the events around us but within ourselves.

It is like learning to discern a frequency and then getting more and more skilled at hearing it even in the midst of a lot of commotion. Our contact with a teacher is one of our primary encounters with the frequency of the teaching. This is why the real teaching has nothing to do with words. So with Rudi, when one moved into his energy field, one wanted to be aware of *its* rhythm.

Learning this kind of awareness is something like playing music with someone else. The first thing you make sure of is that everybody is following the same rhythm. When you first sit down, the initial friction has to do with getting everybody to do so. There is always that momentary uncertainty, regardless of how long the different musicians have played together. You have to feel for the discrepancies between the rhythm of the music and the rhythm you are actually playing. Furthermore, each piece has variations in tempo, even though the fundamental rhythm remains the same. While the tempo is relevant, the primary thing is the rhythm.

As students we want to center and establish ourselves in the rhythm that is the teaching. When we can attune our conscious minds to that rhythm and operate from that field, it doesn't matter where we are or how many thoughts are going through our heads. We are still looking for the basic rhythm. We may find we have to stop over and over again to find it, but this is not a problem. Any musician who is improvising has to keep coming back to the fundamental rhythm. Even when we depart from it for a while, we always come back to it.

In the beginning of our practice we are aware of this rhythm, but our attention is easily distracted by our thoughts and feelings. It takes time and practice to develop the capacity to sustain our awareness of it. We come back to it over and over again, until it becomes almost second nature to override the distractions and return our attention to a deeper focus. This requires, first, the decision to tune into that rhythm; second, the ability to sustain our awareness of it; and third, the determination to function from that awareness.

Yet this is not an effort. It is like loving somebody and wanting to stay in harmony with the fundamental vibration that they are. We learn to transcend our emotional baggage not merely to have more adequate ways of dealing with tension, helpful as this may be in our daily lives. The real aim is to bring ourselves into harmony with this deeper rhythm so that it becomes the point from which we live.

Each of us brings a specific rhythm into the energy field of the teacher. We must learn to transcend this specific rhythm in order to bring ourselves into harmony with the field of the teaching. So when we are in the company of the teacher we try to be quiet and centered within ourselves. From that quiet center we connect to the larger field and begin to feel an exchange of energy. The more deeply we can open, the more deeply the energy penetrates the tensions within us and connects us to ourselves. No words need to be exchanged; a look is enough because the transmission is really heart-to-heart and mind-to-mind.

When we sit with the teacher, our awareness of his or her rhythm emerges from the stillness we first establish within ourselves. We try to catch hold of it and keep hold of it irrespective of its tempo. It is a little bit like catching a wave. The intensification brought about by the experience of that creative energy reorganizes all the structures of our physical bodies, minds, and emotions. We kick up the voltage inside ourselves and become more intense people. But in the process we reduce our own levels of internal resistance and diffusion.

We develop a deeper capacity for concentration and a different order of clarity.

As students we have to be alert at all times to the rhythm of what we are relating to. We have to be capable of changing gears on two levels: first, of catching the rhythm, and then of changing tempo. When we are with the teacher, we are feeling for this rhythm. When we get lost, we look for it again. If our concentration drifts, the first thing we try to pick up on is always the rhythm.

I remember standing in the street outside of Rudi's store for a half hour or forty-five minutes before going in, just attuning myself to the rhythm of what was going on in the store. When I felt some confidence that I was set in it, I would move inside and try to pick up on the tempo. It is in our awareness of this rhythm and its various tempos, along with our capacity to attune ourselves to these, that a powerful unity establishes itself. This unity is something special and wonderful, and it is to be cultivated under every circumstance.

Our awareness of that rhythm will have a tremendous influence on the timing with which we act in our lives and on the attitudes we adopt when we speak. Once we are aware of it, though, it is continuously there for us. It becomes a support and guidance mechanism as we move through our everyday lives and deal with the various difficulties that confront us.

In a very real sense there are so many things about working with energy — about relating from and to it — that are not explainable. There are no exact words with which to talk about the subtleties involved. Therefore, there is no canned answer or cookbook statement I can give for how to do it. What I do think is that as we connect to and participate in it, the understanding comes to us even in the most difficult of situations.

As we cultivate that understanding, a certain purity emerges within us that dissolves our egocentrism and makes our perspective profoundly expansive. We start to experience this unity and stabilize ourselves in it. Then we understand that there is no such thing as an Other and, this being the case, that we serve the whole, the essential reality of the Self.

A Closeness Beyond Distance

As beginning students we talk about energies in time and space. We speak of the transmission of information: about energy flows, interaction, and service. From a more advanced point of view, however, there is no discussion of separation of any kind. Instead, as we refine our awareness of the rhythm of the teaching, there is a shared awareness — a shared, universal experience, in fact — that transcends our individuality. This has no concern for getting ahead or falling behind.

This understanding does not necessarily come easily. A great deal of the inner work we do will express itself in the form of some interaction with a teacher. Through that interaction, our understanding will be tested continuously. This makes it essential for us to be well established in the recognition that there is only one thing. This recognition is what allows us to have a sense of the vitality of that one thing which is, at the same time, the creative energy of our bodies, minds, and emotions, as well as of our individual spirits.

It becomes essential for us to be so attuned to this energy that we understand it also to be manifesting as everybody else around us. Our contact with and service to a teacher are simply the process in which we unite and communicate with that teacher *in* this one spirit. We thereby express our respect for it and our cultivation of the understanding that we experience within that context.

The discussion of rhythm is another way of saying that, in the relationship with the teacher, a kind of merging, or bonding, naturally takes place. It is a bonding, however, in which neither party — especially the teacher — ever loses sight of the fact that both are really merging into the divine. It is a release from bondage rather than a binding to one another. Essentially we recognize and respect the infinite freedom implicit in the creative energy to manifest itself whenever, wherever, and however it wants to.

This may sound idealistic, but if we have any other attitude, it will be a case of our taking the other person for granted. This not only limits that person but, more importantly, it limits us. The idea that if we love somebody, we must set them free has become something of a cliché, which tends to obscure just how important an idea it is. It is not a statement about irresponsibility or a lack of commitment but of profound responsibility and commitment.

It hurts not to set up a chemical bonding. We are forced to overcome our tendency to want to put that bondage in place and go on automatic forever. Still, the communion that takes place when we are deeply open is a communion in divine consciousness that frees everybody from bondage and binding. Our own bindings will loosen in the process, and we will feel some anxiety as we recognize the profound uncertainty that naturally accompanies the condition of absolute freedom. It hurts. We may even have a few panic attacks because of it. Yet in our relationship with the teacher, we do not want to establish relationships that are actually dependencies. Rather we want to establish a ground in which mature relationships can develop.

The attitude of a teacher and a student toward this relationship is quite different. The teacher is an available resource. The challenge that the student faces is to develop and extend that availability as he or she absorbs the information that exists within that resource. The role of a teacher in our lives then becomes the opportunity to discover and achieve a state of detachment. In that state we cultivate the simplicity, clarity, focus, discipline, and courage that enable us to become established in our introspection. In this way we become established in our quest to participate deeply in the source of our own, and all, awareness.

Some kind of maturity can and should evolve in the context of this relationship. Certainly we will find that, as in any relationship, the distance we feel changes. Sometimes we feel extremely close, while at other times we may feel more distant. In one sense, these are simply experiences that are normal. Yet in this kind of relationship the distinction also has no real meaning because closeness and distance with the individual become irrelevant. It is the rhythm of the teaching in which we want to participate.

At this level, therefore, closeness can be defined differently. As beginning students we think of "close" as meaning that we can talk and say whatever we want, share whatever concerns we have, and so on. Being close means we have a forum for all this. Closeness, however, now means something quite different. In my experience with Rudi, for example, I almost never got to talk to him. There was little need to, because conversation was not the point of the relationship. At this level neither talking nor sharing our individual points of view, or any other aspect of concrete interaction, is the point. There may be some operational interaction, but even that is pretty simple.

Real closeness is our participation in this rhythm. Real closeness is also quiet. It is, after all, hard to talk about awareness, especially as it has no thought content to it. It has no mind as we usually understand mind, nor does it have emotional content as we ordinarily experience our emotions. It does, however, have the experience of what I call a sense of total well-being. This is a simple thing. We could say that in this closeness, the real transmission takes place. In fact, though, even the discussion of transmission is eliminated because the unity that is established goes beyond separation. In a real way, what need is there to transmit anything?

This level of practice has nothing to do with individuality in the slightest. It has nothing to do with having a close personal relationship with the teacher or a distant one. It has nothing to do with the mastery of ideas or with our capacity to articulate them. Notions such as I'm a good person, I'm a bad person, I am liked, I am not liked, life is fair, life is not fair, and so on and endlessly so forth, have nothing to do with anything. We understand, instead, that there is a dynamic at work here that extends us and pulls us back. It extends our experience and contracts it.

This requires some personal, inner experience and some years of observation. However, reflecting on those personal experiences allows them to become part of our data bank. The extent to which we maintain our balance through these various experiences as they unfold each successive wave is the extent to which we are expanded and uplifted naturally, without having to think about it. We may have to attend to a few details and do a little work, but these things, also, just happen.

In a certain way, the whole process of the student-teacher relationship is the mutual recognition, or reunification, of the fundamental Self which is the essence of all. This is why it is not exactly a bonding but rather a liberation from our individual, limited sense of who and what we are. The relationship itself is a force that functions to change the total pattern of our creative expression.

The human teacher is basically a servant to those people who have expressed their wish to experience universal integration. He or she is a resource, available in service to the same. What this really means, though, is that in serving the cause of universal integration, he or she is serving not another person but the dismantling of the ego. The energy of the teacher is transmitted to the student, and the student's own creative energy is aroused, thereby giving him or her direct experience of the pulsation of Life Itself within. This has the effect of dissolving all our concepts and thought constructs, and of establishing our minds in the awareness of our true nature.

Ultimately the teacher is that highest state of knowledge about the nature of our individuality, the process of Life Itself, and the relationship between the two. To be totally devoted to serving that knowledge and truth is what liberates a human being. In this way the teacher is the means.

MEDITATION

By uniting with the great lake — the infinite reservoir
of Divine Power — one has the experience of the
Supreme I-consciousness which is the generative source
of all mantras.

— SHIVA SUTRAS

In the discussion of anavopaya, we talked about meditation as a set of practices that we do. In shaktopaya it is not that
we stop doing any of these practices; on the contrary, they
always remain the basis of our inner work from the beginning
to the end. At the same time, our experience of them
changes. It is like riding a bicycle. At first we have to pay
attention all the time just to keep our balance and avoid falling
off. Eventually, however, the techniques involved become
more or less second nature.

It is true that when the road gets especially bumpy, we
have to bring our conscious attention back to what it takes to
keep our balance, but for the most part, we stop thinking
about this part of the whole thing. Instead, we become able to
look around us and enjoy the scenery. In shaktopaya what we
see when we look around at the scenery is the energy of spanda
as it expresses itself in all things.

The Trika thinkers were extraordinarily sophisticated in
their descriptions of the phases of practice. They showed, for
example, how a given technique starts out as part of anavopaya
and in the course of practice shifts over into the awareness of
shaktopaya and, eventually, into that of shambhavopaya. This,
essentially, is the content of the *Vijnanabhairava*, an ancient text
that is basically a practitioner's manual of techniques and
descriptions of shifts in awareness.

In our own discussion we are going to look at two ways
in which the awareness of anavopaya emerges into the awareness of shaktopaya: first, with the discussion of mantra, and,
second, with a discussion of the pause between two breaths.
Both begin as techniques and, therefore, as part of anavopaya;

both translate into the possibility of an extraordinary awareness of the pulsation of spanda.

MANTRA, MATRIKA, AND THE MIND

This is the supreme joy, the supreme medicine, the
supreme guru, whose mantra is: That thou art; thou
art That.

— NITYANANDA

For the beginning student first learning to practice meditation, there are a lot of things to think about: becoming aware of our breath, the chakras, flow, and a sense of presence. As we have seen, much of our attention is taken up with becoming at ease with the necessary techniques and with everything we have to do to quiet our minds. We learn to relax in order to get at a simple, undistracted awareness. We open ourselves and become sensitive to the dynamic reality that underlies our bodies, minds, and emotions. Having that experience, we learn to remain focused on it.

As advanced students we do the same things but notice different things about them. As the nature of our inner work becomes more refined and subtle, our experience of it gradually changes. What is the gist of this change? It parallels the shift in our experience of the guru: Our focus moves from technique and effort, or the level of individual experience, to an awareness of the energy, or vibration.

In order to talk about how this happens, the Trika masters explored two important areas of experience: the nature of the human mind and the nature of language. They looked at how both of these are part of the dynamic contraction of spanda, and at how they play a part in covering over our awareness of the highest reality. They also looked at how our inner work reverses this process. This took them into the study of mantra. We will look at these topics both with regard to the observations of the Trika masters and our own experience of them.

The Nature of the Mind

Mind is the root of bondage and liberation, of good and evil, of sin and holiness.

— NITYANANDA

In the West the discussion of the mind usually falls under the heading of psychology, and there are as many ways of talking about it as there are different schools of thought. The mind has been studied by scientists as a chemical and neurological part of us. Seen as the part of us that enables us to know, the mind has been explored in its relation to different ways of learning. It has also been discussed as consisting of different components, the specifics of which vary depending on whose orientation you are working with. Yet all these approaches have something in common. Each of them grows out of an understanding of what a human being has the potential to be. Each is connected with therapeutic strategies that aim to bring about the fulfillment of that potential.

In India the study of the mind has been part of a greater concern for refining human awareness to the most subtle degree possible. This awareness has been understood to go beyond certain aspects of the mind. The people who explored the mind from this perspective did so with an interest in what aspects of the mind get in the way of this awareness and what aspects support our work to bring it about.

The mind as a whole they called *chitta*. This is our individual consciousness, or the mind of the individual. It consists of three aspects, known as *buddhi*; *ahamkar*, or the ego; and *manas*. The first of these aspects, buddhi, can be called our ascertaining intelligence. It is our capacity for ascertainment, decision, and intelligent will. It is our higher mind, or wisdom. Buddhi is the intuitive aspect of our awareness by which we awaken to the truth about ourselves.

Buddhi is farsighted. It is what kicks in when we see the big picture. It is not concerned with either pleasure or pain but only with truth. In the face of every difficulty and complexity, buddhi is the part of us that recognizes our own and everyone else's highest best interest. If we have ever made decisions on this basis, we have drawn on the part of us that is buddhi. Nityananda called it our subtle discrimination and spiritual discernment.

One reason why buddhi can see things in the light of the big picture is that it is not concerned with that famous question that so often preoccupies us: "What's going to happen to me?" That is the job of the second aspect of chitta known as ahamkar or, as we are more used to calling it, the ego. The ego is the mechanism in us that draws together what we experience as "I," in the narrowest sense. It is what thinks in terms of "I," "me," and "mine."

The ego sees things in terms of the small picture. It is what identifies with our bodies, needs, wants, and desires as individuals. It is always asking variations on the mantra of ignorance: "How will I get ahead and how do I keep from falling behind? How can I win, and how to avoid losing?" It is the ego that says, in countless ways, "Don't hurt me!" and tries to run away from pain. So it is also the part of us that continuously tries first to define the lines and boundaries of our lives and then to hold them in place. Ordinarily the ego is our basic operating system. After all, think about how much time and energy we put into figuring out how to further what we perceive to be our own interests, whether in terms of our work or our relationships, as elaborations of our biological imperatives to eat and reproduce.

The third aspect of our individual consciousness is called manas. This is the part of us that reacts to the impressions and data gathered by our senses and that cooperates with the senses in building our perceptions. When I sometimes refer to the mind as a pattern-recognition mechanism, I am talking about manas. From these perceptions manas builds up images, concepts, intentions, and especially thought-constructs, known as *vikalpas*.

Like the ego, manas is limited and gets us into trouble by directing our attention outward. Manas reaches for pleasure and avoids pain; it therefore entangles us in thoughts of wanting one thing or another. So manas has to do with the gross expression of our minds through thoughts, concepts, and feelings. It is the function of buddhi to discriminate among these thoughts, concepts, and feelings to discern their meaning.

When Rudi used to talk about the mind as the slayer of the soul, he was referring to manas, the grosser aspect of chitta. Sometimes he would talk about the higher mind, in order to make a distinction. In the field of our experience, manas forms patterns out of our perceptions. The ego, ahamkar, appropriates these in relation to its sense of "I." The intellect, buddhi, is the bridge between chitta as a whole and infinite consciousness.

In reflecting on the nature of the mind, the Trika masters were also interested in vikalpas, or thought-constructs. They observed that a vikalpa is the means by which the mind differentiates one thing from another as it divides reality into particulars. Each vikalpa has an inclusive aspect: It selects things and groups them into categories, like chairs or dogs, at the same time as it has ways of describing differences between things in the same category, like sofas and benches. Each vikalpa also has an exclusive aspect: When it includes a certain thing in one category, it excludes everything else. The category of chairs does not include dogs.

Vikalpas can refer to all the things in the external world. They can also refer to all the things we imagine that have no correspondence in material reality. A bird that gives milk, for example, *is* a thought-construct, even if no such thing really exists. At the same time, the idea does have some correspondence to material reality, in that birds as well as creatures that give milk both exist; it is our capacity for vikalpas that joins the two. In either case we are still talking about the most contracted dimension of reality. This is the level of experience to which the vikalpas correspond.

We could say that vikalpas are the tags we put on things to tell us how to respond to them. They always describe a reality of subjects and objects, because we always have a thought *about* something else, some "other." So vikalpas are an integral aspect of dualistic thinking. Indeed, vikalpas *are* dualistic by nature, as is all thought.

This means that vikalpas obstruct our seeing reality from the perspective of the biggest picture. We identify with our thoughts, we assume that reality corresponds to them, and it rarely occurs to us that anything might be otherwise. When we think, "I am happy, I am sad, I am thin, I am fat," and so on, we take these ideas to be true about ourselves. Moreover, all these constructs get colored by judgments and values. We assume that being happy and thin are good, and being sad and fat are bad. Then, instead of questioning how our perceptions get structured in these ways, we live according to our judgments, as though they were facts of life.

We forget that as biological entities we are essentially colonies of cells in which each cell is constantly communicating its own program. The energy transmitted between cells has in every case a vibrational, or sound, component. So we could say that the cells are all talking to each other all the time. Our thoughts are primarily the net effect of the different vibrations generated by the different cells functioning in our systems.

Broadly speaking, these vibrations group themselves according to the perceived needs to eat and reproduce. We are constantly evaluating everything in terms of whether it supports or obstructs these biological imperatives. Our thought constructs sustain our identification with the ego, preventing us from recognizing the Self. The intent of our inner work is to release us from the bonds of these concepts and constructs, to allow us to see the vitality of Life Itself as it is.

Matrika: The Nature of Language

> *It is the Mother who is not understood, the power of sound, that is the basis of limited knowledge.*

> — SHIVA SUTRAS

The Meaning of Matrika

As they looked at the ways in which the energy of Life Itself crystallizes into our experience as individuals, the Trika masters found they could not discuss chitta without also looking at its relation to language. After all, language shapes our thoughts, and we use it much of the time to express ourselves.

What interested these people about language was the gap they found between the words we use and the reality we are talking about. This led them to examine just how language, along with chitta, obscures our awareness of the highest reality. This was a variation on the discussion of spanda. I say "variation" because in relation to language, these masters focused on pulsation, or vibration, as sound. The great science, and the highest formulation of Trika Yoga that emerged as a result, was the science of sound.

The discussion of the tattvas, as we have seen, is an attempt to interrelate everything from living forms, mind, thought, and matter as expressions of the pulsation of Life Itself. They pointed out that the subtle vibration of infinite consciousness, which we have already discussed as spanda, is the foundation of all our mental structures.

The Trika masters also called this subtle pulsation *matrika*. In Sanskrit *matr* refers to "mother," while *ka* is added to a word to show that the thing is unknown, or not understood. Therefore, *matri-ka* means the mother that is not properly known or understood. It is a way of saying that we do not ordinarily understand the true nature of language or the source from which it springs.

The Unfolding of Sound

Just as the Trika Yoga practitioners had developed the thirty-six tattvas to describe the self-expression of the energy, they also spelled out a series of steps by which the subtlest resonance, or matrika, contracts into spoken words. Nityananda expressed this more simply, saying, "Does sound arise from the universe, or does the universe arise from sound? Effect from cause or cause from effect? The universe arises from sound; from sound, form arises, and all things that have form."

The Trika Yoga thinkers worked out four phases in this process. They said that first of all, from one quiet, pure awareness, the pulsation called spanda arises as the desire of the

Absolute to express itself. The potentiality to manifest is present, but nothing has yet emerged. This phase is called *paravak*, or the highest word.

The resonance of this phase is called *nada*, or the Om-sound. This is the high-pitched sound we hear when we become quiet and that, as we become quieter still, we hear more and more. The poet Kabir refers to it as the divine symphony. From nada, the whole world has come forth. This is the fundamental resonance, or word, pulsating in us and in all things. It is the pulsation from which all language originates, even as it permeates all language as its essence. It is the word of God.

The second phase is called *pashyanti*, a word whose Sanskrit root means "to see." This is the first showing, or seeing, of what has the potential to emerge. It is like when you drop a rock in water. There is a lag between when the rock hits the water and when the vibration starts to spread out from that point.

Paravak is a little bit like the very moment when the rock and the water meet. This contact sets up a center of turbulence. The difference is that in the infinite, every single point is a center of the turbulence. Pashyanti is the impulse to move out from those centers. It does not represent a fully articulated event itself. Instead, it represents the potential, or capacity, for articulation to take place. At that stage, there is still no differentiation. Everything is present, but nothing has expressed itself as actual sound.

It is in the next stage that this extreme subtlety moves to a point where the reality of sound is about to emerge. This vitality, which is the power of self-realization, knowledge, and action, starts to coalesce as the *power* to burst out in song. Notice that it is not actually the song itself but the inspiration or feeling behind it. *This* is the power of matrika. I would point out, in this regard, that the aspect of reality that was least interesting to the Trika thinkers was the concrete one with which we interact every day. Rather they were interested in the energy as a process and in how it gathered itself up to manifest.

In their exploration of the next phase of sound, they investigated the multiple nuances of vibration they encountered on all levels of reality. This phase they called *madhyama*. These most basic vibrations they referred to as "letters" because, just as letters of the alphabet represent the sounds out of which we compose our speech and express our reality, so the vibrations of the ultimate come together to express themselves as all of manifest reality.

These "letters," of course, are not simply symbols for sounds the way the English-language ABC is. Instead, they refer to living vibrations that, as they manifest, have a sound component to them. We could say that the universe is nothing but a network of letters — a network that is the sound-body of God. In the same way, every human being is made up of such letters. Even the mind is nothing but these.

The letters of the Sanskrit language came forth based on this understanding of vibration. They were an attempt to approximate, in gross form, the subtlety of these pulsations and their interaction. According to the theory of matrika, the Sanskrit letters represent all the possible sounds available in the universe. They are the subvibrations out of which we form words: the mechanisms by which we structure our experience, classify our thoughts and feelings, and organize the connections that make up our individualized field of consciousness.

The essence of any sound is a vibration at a particular frequency. Matrika is the totality of these vibrations, which give rise to all form, all feeling, all thoughts, words and actions. All language is based on matrika. In every aspect of our lived-through experience, this is the reality we are dealing with. Matrika is the vibration implicit in consciousness that is the *basis* of thought. Matrika thus refers not to the character of the individual but to our articulation of the divine.

All of us generate feelings from within ourselves. Some are self-generated, while others arise in response to the medium in which we find ourselves. The self-to-self events are what we experience as inspiration, or sometimes intuition, while the responses to outside feelings are what we experience as reactions. In either case these subtle feelings arise and organize themselves as the concepts, or vikalpas, we talked about earlier, and from these concepts, thoughts come forth. For example, as we become entangled in and identified with observing who likes us and who doesn't, who said a nice thing to us and who said something mean, the interaction between these feelings, the vikalpas that arise from them, and the vibration of the environment in response, come together and crystallize as an identity that we buy into.

Then as victims of our own feelings, thoughts, and emotions, we experience unhappiness, pain, and suffering, and extend the same throughout the world. Finally we conclude that the bottom line of our lives is that something is fundamentally wrong with us. This is bondage. It happens only because we don't know any better. We remain unaware that the whole range of feelings we have is implicit within the existence of matrika, as is our capacity to recognize and articulate them.

If we listen only to words, we don't get the real idea of what is being said at all. This is because words alone fragment reality into what seem like separate entities and experiences, and suggest that reality is many instead of one. As I said earlier, all thought is dualistic, and words are what structure our thoughts. Thus words, in and of themselves, are quite limited. All of this is related to matrika, insofar as words are formed from the letters, or vibrations, of matrika. In its relation to words and language, therefore, matrika forms the basis of all limited knowledge.

One of the most extended, crystallized levels of this whole process is the fourth phase of sound, or actual speech, known as *vaikari*. Our communication takes place in part through the vibrations we group into the words we pass back and forth between us. Vaikari is a way of discussing the densest form of speech while at the same time showing its unbroken connection to the most subtle resonance of paravak.

The power of speech is nothing but the kundalini energy pulsating within us, interacting with itself, and evolving from within itself the networks of vibration. These we string together into the thoughts, concepts, and feelings that we then speak, and that have great impact in our lives.

There is thus no real separation between any feeling we have, or word we say, and the universal consciousness of which we are a part. In fact, it is this medium of consciousness that allows us to communicate in the first place. If we had nothing profoundly in common, no connection or understanding would be possible.

The Power of Speech and Words

Everybody makes more or less the same sounds. Different cultures organize them in different ways to communicate the concepts related both to their experience and environment and to the time and place in which they exist. Still, among all people, sound plays a fundamentally important role. The power of sound is related to our very survival as a species.

The power of even common speech is great, and it is one that in every way molds and shapes our experience. If you walk into a store and say, "I would like an apple," it is quite likely (unless you have gone into a plumbing supply store) that you will be given an apple. The power of speech is such that it can manifest what is imagined and wanted.

The different thoughts and feelings that manifest from us as words and actions have their concrete imprint on every aspect of our experience and on the experience of those with whom we interact. In this sense, words — vibrations and sounds — are our power. For example, the power of our speech inspires everything from hatred, bitterness, jealousy, and every kind of misfortune and pain, to a sense of total well-being, pleasure, and satisfaction. Because of words, we are constantly having our feelings hurt and hurting those of others, and getting entangled in a web of uncertainty. We experience doubt, fear, disappointment, and unhappiness.

If I look at someone and say, "You idiot, stop that!" it produces one immediate reaction. If, on the other hand, I say, "I love you very much," this generates a different and equally immediate reaction. This is the potential of speech to create antagonism or harmony, to establish a vibration.

Furthermore, although we may not think about it that deeply, that same power of speech within us is what also enables us to evolve a sense of self, or identity. It is what allows us to classify and understand who we are and what we want — what our purpose is both in a big way and in thousands of little ways.

At the same time, the words we use to communicate with one another are not in any way separate from the energy of Life Itself; rather they are implicit within it. They are the way we symbolize the features of the vibration we share. Through them we awaken a deeper part of the shared experience in which we participate, and arouse a shared awareness of the network of vibrations by which we are essentially united.

We use words to make another person aware of the features of our shared experience in order to *make* it just that: a shared experience. We thereby attempt to extend our energy field. From a deeper perspective, words are thus the mechanisms by which the Self intends to awaken Itself.

That we take this for granted doesn't make it any less powerful. Try going to a country where almost no one speaks your language. You will find at once that what you know as the power of your language suddenly becomes fairly impotent. Then it is easier to see something of the impact it has on your life.

Words have tremendous generative power, and yet rarely are we careful about how we use them. What extends from words is action. Thus we must recognize the lasting impact of our words and actions on the patterns of creative energy of our lives. Depending upon what we express, we either create an obstruction to the whole program or a vehicle that will tap the deepest part of our potential and allow it to come forth.

Matrika as Our Misunderstanding

The creative energy of Life Itself is the source of all creation and the manifestation of joy. At the same time, it is also the greatest source of our misunderstanding about our own nature. This is why matrika means "the mother who is not understood," or "unknown mother." It is the hidden source of every form and substance, the mother of all creation.

Creation here means all that we experience. It refers to the notion that matrika is the source of ideas, concepts, and language on the one hand, and on the other hand, material reality as it unfolds through time, space, and the different stages of what we call condensation. Sometimes this is personified as the goddess Vyomesh, or "she who regurgitates the whole universe."

In the *Shiva Sutras* it says that as long as a person is under the influence of matrika — that is, does not understand its nature — then matrika is a source of bondage. Then he or she will suffer in the currents of the stream of existence. This is because the play of matrika in the realm of time and space gives rise to differentiated objects and, in the inner realm, to the play of feelings and thoughts. It is because of matrika that we experience one thing as different from another.

It is because of matrika that our vision of the divine is obscured. When we are entangled in the information provided by our senses, or when we are caught up in the misunderstanding of ourselves as limited creatures separate from God and from the source of Life, we experience ourselves as powerless. We allow ourselves to give in to frustration, and succumb to tensions and mental confusion. When these things happen, we are under the domination of matrika.

The crystallized form of our individuality causes us to react to the feelings and thoughts that arise within us, limiting our horizon to these feelings. Because we don't understand the nature of our feelings and their relation to the Absolute, our feelings of being good or bad — as well as our perceptions of pleasure and pain of every kind — all act to limit us. This gives our thoughts and feelings power over us. We don't understand them as spontaneous, creative expressions emerging from a deeper level of awareness within us. We don't recognize that they are nothing but changes of frequency in the constant vibration that we are, or that we ourselves can change the channel.

Instead, our perception tells us that there are beginnings and endings to things; that there even is such as a thing as time and space. We take it for granted that there are linear relationships between these supposed beginnings and endings when, in fact, our senses receive only a portion of the pulsation and experience only a small part of it. As an analogy, if we were raised in a valley we might think of it as the whole universe. Only when we stand high on one of the mountains do we see the broader perspective.

When we do not understand the power of words and their ultimate source, we are bound by these words and their meanings, and by ideas and concepts. We become the creations of our words. Only when we are aware of their nature can they become a real tool, a means with no particular meaning beyond their efficacy *as* tools. Therefore, to attain the awareness of matrika is the heart of the primary strategy of shaktopaya: mantra.

Mantra

The mind that reflects on mantra becomes mantra.

— SHIVA SUTRAS

Mantra in Beginning Practice

Man, the Sanskrit root of the word "mantra," means "to think over deeply, to consider or contemplate, to ruminate." *Tra* implies that this contemplation, at the very least, brings safe passage through worldly experience while, at its fullest, it brings about a real awakening. In India many different mantras were developed centuries ago as part of a wide range of treatment strategies. It was thought, for example, that the repetition of a mantra was essential for healing to occur. In some cases, mantras exist for quasi-magical purposes, to alter or reorganize the nature of experience. People repeated various mantras to receive benefits or to develop spiritual powers. In their deepest sense, however, mantra brings a person into the experience of the Absolute.

At the most basic level, a mantra is a word with some resonance that is, in some way, sacred or symbolic. It is the individuated syllable or phrase we say with the intention of reaching or recognizing the highest state of Self-awareness. At this level of our practice, mantra is the effort we make in the context of our limited individuality, and it therefore has to do with the phase of anavopaya. At this stage we may experience it as a kind of prayer or as the expression of some desire. The repetition of a mantra helps us focus our attention and trains our concentration. So mantra functions to support a steady mind in the practice of meditation.

The idea behind this is that if you have a busy mind, it is better to be involved in the repetition of mantra than to have your thoughts drive you all over town. Our options make themselves clear, just as the choices we are called upon to make show themselves in due time. Thus to quiet the mind through mantra gives us an alternative to wondering or plotting about our various options. This is one of the practical benefits of mantra practice.

In many traditions, the practice of mantra was preliminary to the experience of meditation with a teacher. Students passed through stages of training in which they spent years memorizing and practicing different mantras along with the gestures particular to each of the various ceremonies. They did this just to arrive at the point where they were able to sustain the experience of working directly with a teacher.

In other words, mantra was intended to help a person deepen his or her awareness to the point where he or she could work effectively with a teacher. In this sense, it was seen as a process of purification. In the Trika system, however, contact with a teacher through whom one received shaktipat brought about the same effect. Then the whole preliminary stage of preparation was not thought to be necessary.

For the Trika thinkers, any discussion of mantra was really a discussion of the pulsation of Life Itself, or of spanda. On the individual level, one of the ways this pulsation articulates itself is as our breath. By becoming aware of our breathing, we gradually become aware of the vibration of the great mantra, that of Life Itself.

To borrow from something the osteopath Ann Wales once said to me, the bones, or structure, of our practice consist of the breath. The chakras, flow, and Presence we discussed earlier are all important, but breath is at the center. For that matter, breathing is the only constant part of our every experience. Twenty-one thousand and six hundred times a day, we breath whether we want to or not. Fortunately this does not depend on the state of our individual consciousness but is an involuntary function that depends upon the fluctuation of the energy within the cerebrospinal fluid. The more we train ourselves to be aware of our breath, the more we become aware of the energy that supports it, and of the power that underlies *that*.

Ultimately, a real mantra requires the transmission of the breath from the teacher to the student. The life force, or the energy — this is the real initiation. Essentially, we don't care what the particular mantra is. The particulars are fundamentally irrelevant. Any mantra upon which you focus your mind has, as its subtle essence, a vibration to which the repetition is intended to attune you.

When you receive that mantra in direct transmission from a teacher, it is really the resonance of the teacher's awareness that is being conveyed to you, not simply a word or a syllable to repeat. This is also why the explanation of mantra must be oral. You can read about mantras in a book, but unless you understand them as vibration — indeed, unless you receive them as a vibration — you will get only limited benefit without the flash of insight into what mantra is really all about. It will then take you years to figure out what to do with it. Mantra is therefore one of the principle reasons why the guru is the means.

Mantra in Advanced Practice

In terms of refining our awareness of the energy, the main strategy of shaktopaya is mantra. Mantra, on one level, consists of words or letters — the gross vibrations of speech, or vaikari. At the same time, as we saw in the discussion of matrika, the essence of all language and words is nothing but creative energy, the vibration of pure awareness itself.

This means that the spanda principle of expansion and contraction is the substratum of all mantras. Conscious energy constitutes the life of a mantra; mantras derive their power from spanda, and subside back into it. The reality of the Self is the secret of all mantras.

In Trika Yoga this becomes both a philosophical statement and a practice involving the use of words in realizing the ultimate cosmic principle. If the science of matrika is the essence of all the Tantras, it is also the essence of mantra. From this science the theory and practice of mantra have emerged as a strategy for changing our own vibration.

In general the point of any mantra practice is to develop within ourselves an awareness of the fundamental ground of all differentiation that is spanda; to attune ourselves to that which supports sound, which is also spanda; and to become established in that which is beyond every kind of differentiation.

The practice of repeating mantras was instituted as a means of penetrating our different thoughts and feelings, much as the close scrutiny of matter by physicists has allowed us to penetrate the appearance of form and solidity. Mantra practice frees us from the various experiences of contraction in which we become entangled, and focuses our attention so that our dualistic thoughts become stabilized in the awareness of a deeper resonance. Then we can rise out of our mental turmoil and confusion any time we desire, and establish ourselves in a higher state.

For the beginning student mantra refers to the repetition of a syllable, but as we practice we must not confuse the recited mantra with the internal mantra, which is not a recitation. As we understand this, mantra eventually becomes an intense awareness and, therefore, an intense degree of reflection or concentration. In the thirteenth-century text the *Mahartha-manjari*, for example, it is not repetition but awareness itself that is mantra.

The essence of the theory of mantra is that vibration is nothing more than the highest creative power, functioning in two ways: first, as *bijas*, or seeds; second, as matrices, or networks. Bijas are vibrations that are extremely pure and simple. As mantras, they have one syllable. Matrices are seed vibrations that have been joined into words or phrases. Mantra thus has both a philosophical substance and a rhythmical, vibrational content.

Mantra practice is important in the advanced stages of our work because it becomes the experience of resonance in an infinite field. The secret of all mantras is the communion of the individual mind with the supreme, divine I-consciousness, which includes within itself the universe. Mantra awakens our awareness of the Self and releases us from the bondage of *samsara*, the stream of experience.

Earlier I said that the guru is the means, and that we deepen our work with the guru to the degree that we become aware of him or her as a field of energy. Another way of saying this is that the guru is established in a highly refined awareness of the vibration of mantra. This makes both the words and presence of the guru — his or her energy field — expressions of that vibration.

To say that the guru teaches the essential truth of mantra refers not to any verbal instruction about mantra. Rather it means that our very contact with the guru conveys to us the potency of mantra. This is the essence of shaktipat. In this way the guru teaches us the mystery of matrika, the secret of the vital breath of Life Itself.

The Mantra That Repeats Itself

Most people are not particularly aware of their breathing even though it goes on all the time. It may be unrhythmic, shaped and structured by the stresses and strains held in the body, and we may never notice. Yet our awareness of our breath is one of the most powerful vehicles we have for entering into a deeper awareness and for changing our state.

In the discussion of matrika I said that there is a resonance that underlies all sound, called nada, or the Om-sound. This vibration has no beginning and no end, so it is spoken of as uncaused and ceaseless. It is known as the unstruck sound, not uttered by anything. It is completely self-generated, yet no one articulates it, nor can anything prevent it. It is the source of all sound and of the very breath of every living creature.

As beginning students we learn to sit down in meditation and pay attention to the rhythm of our breathing, focusing at first on the inbreath and the outbreath. One reason we do this is to quiet our minds, because there is a direct relationship between the breath and the state of the mind. At the same time, our awareness of our breath is a gateway to an awareness of the unstruck sound.

Initially we learn a simple mantra to accompany the breath. As we inhale we mentally say the syllable *soh*; as we exhale, we mentally say the syllable *hahm* — *soham* — or what is known as the *hamsa* mantra. One syllable represents inhalation; the other, exhalation. So whether we are actually repeating the syllables themselves or not, we are repeating this mantra automatically with every round of breath. We do this 21,600 times a day. This form of mantra repetition, or *japa*, is known as *ajapa-japa*, the repetition that goes on spontaneously, without effort.

In the practice of Trika Yoga, as we train ourselves to be aware of our breath, we gradually also become aware of more subtle aspects of this mantra. This is not surprising. Rudi used to say that it was a source of great strength for him to do a simple exercise for a long period of time, allowing it to go deeper and deeper. He felt that basic work of this kind was the foundation of spirituality and that such elementary exercises afforded us the possibility to refine our awareness to an extraordinarily subtle degree.

As we refine our awareness of this particular exercise, gradually we notice that it is not exactly we who are doing the breathing. This is not only because our breathing happens involuntarily but because within our physical breath there is an even more subtle pulsation going on. When we begin to practice meditation, for example, we notice that the base of our spine rocks gently forward when we exhale and backward when we inhale. This subtle rocking motion moves up the spinal column and is related to a fluctuation of the energy within the cerebrospinal fluid.

If we really tune into the waves of this energy, we become aware of what I call the breath within the breath. By becoming quiet we can awaken to that vibration within ourselves and participate in it. We discover that it has a way of coalescing as energy, coming to a stillpoint, and shifting to release into a more open state. Gradually we have the experience not of repeating the mantra but of the mantra repeating us; we experience ourselves not as breathing, exactly, but as being breathed.

The Changing of Frequency

I would like to return for a moment to some further considerations about the mind and the implications for mantra practice. I have thought for some time that the mind is not centered in the brain but that it permeates the whole body. By this I mean not just that it is linked to the nervous system but that the body and the mind are fundamentally one thing. The nervous system is just part of the framework, as are the bones, with both existing to support the mind. Likewise, the immune system is a part of the mind. So, for example, the more open the mind, the healthier the body.

The mind extends throughout the entire system and is not separable from it. This suggests that as we modify the rhythm of the body, the mind is affected, and vice versa. The various emotional states we experience have, at their core, different vibrations, each of which has a different effect on us. This is like our experience of music: Rock has one vibration, while classical music has another. If we listen to one kind, it makes us feel heavy and melancholy; if we listen to another, we may feel more light-hearted and at ease.

Likewise, every one of us has a fundamental vibration that we not only carry around with us, but that we *are*. In the beginning, this vibration is essentially an expression of our limitation. It is the sum of all the various strains, traumas, and stresses that we carry within us. It is something like trying to ring a bell packed with cotton. There is a vibration but it is muffled, muted, and dull.

The effect of mantra repetition as a practice is literally to change the vibration that we are. Some people also argue that it brings us to the point where we can begin to experience the pure stage of vibration present within us all the time. My own experience is also that if we are working with a teacher, we can leap over the intermediate stage and get right to the direct heart of it.

When we understand this system well and learn how to alter its frequency in even small ways, we find we can change the shape of all the experiences around us. The next time you are sitting in meditation and working with a mantra, as you concentrate on the different levels of vibration, notice the change that happens throughout your entire sympathetic nervous system. Instead of directing your attention to your lungs or your legs, feel what is going on in your system as a whole. If you can feel a change happening in just that short period of time, is it not reasonable to think that, over time, a change might happen that would have a profound effect on you as a whole — on how you express yourself, and on what your life attracts?

The Mind as the Root of Freedom

The first sutra in the anavopaya section of the *Shiva Sutras* says that chitta, or the complex of buddhi, ahamkar (the ego), and manas, is what we usually experience as our individual selves. This, as we have talked about, is why it is said that the mind is the root of our confusion. We have looked at some of the ways that our minds' involvement with thought constructs and language further reinforces this confusion.

We have also seen that mantra practice serves as a way of changing the resonance of the mind, bringing it into attunement with the deeper pulsation of Life Itself, which brings us to a paradox: The mind is both the entity to be quieted and the means of quieting it. Nityananda used to say that the mind is the root of both bondage and freedom. Like everything, it cuts both ways. It can be a source either of resistance or support to our inner work.

It is not a support when it is locked into the vikalpas with which we usually think about ourselves: "I am weak, ignorant, and limited, and there is something other than myself that I lack." But if thought constructs are part of the very nature of the mind, then how can the mind get around that kind of dualistic thinking? Only if there is one vikalpa that cuts through every dualistic thought, one vikalpa that identifies us with the highest reality — only if the mind can absorb that thought so deeply that it sees everything from that perspective — then, it is possible.

This vikalpa occurs in the idea that "I" and the "Self" are the same: "I am the Self." This is basically the meaning expressed by the hamsa mantra. *Aham* in Sanskrit means "I," and *sah* means "That" in the sense of Shiva, or the essential Self. So this mantra, in addition to establishing us in an increasingly deeper awareness of our breath, also establishes us in the nondualistic awareness that I and the Self are neither separate nor different.

For the mind to experience this it must be quiet. This kind of quiet is called the state of *nirvikalpa samadhi*, a perfectly quiet mind without (*nir-*) vikalpas, or thought constructs. It is this experience that has its own purifying impact on us. By sitting in this awareness and by re-examining it over and over again, we come to a clearer recognition of what it is and of how to stay in it.

We realize, too, that this takes us beyond the bonds of matrika. It is not as if we need an antidote to matrika. There *is* no antidote, exactly, because it is not bad in the first place. While it is both a tension and an obstruction for those who do not understand it, those who *do* understand experience it as the source underlying all multiplicity.

To be liberated from the tyranny of matrika is to be freed from the tyranny of ideas and concepts. It is to be established in the direct, clear experience of the breath of Life. This is the freedom of matrika. When her mystery is realized, she is the source of our awakening.

In shaktopaya, by becoming aware of everything as energy and by striving to attune ourselves to finer and finer frequencies of that energy, we create within ourselves the capacity to relate to all frequencies. An understanding of matrika is the basis by which all real spiritual capacities manifest. This is not an intellectual understanding but rather an intuitive grasp, or contact, that allows us to be aware of all the energies functioning in a particular event.

This contact also allows us to attune ourselves to these energies so that we can be aware of all the separate frequencies happening within one complex circumstance. We are then able to tune into both the finest as well as the heaviest frequencies. We sometimes do the former as a way of participating in and altering the structure and frequency of that vibration, thereby modifying the structure of our experience.

Various texts point out that when a person attains the understanding of matrika, then all self-discipline, austerity, inner work, and joy merge perfectly. All of life unfolds before us as an expression of the immense vitality, love, and joy of our own inner Self, that supreme divine I-consciousness that shimmers within each of us.

A person established in this highest awareness would say, "Everything is the Self. There is nothing different from it and never any separation from God." All that is, is the play of God's creative energy. Thus, which part of it is not perfection? Which part is not beautiful or lacks joy? Everything is seen as God's grace.

The Mind as Mantra

The first sutra in the shaktopaya section of the *Shiva Sutras* says, "The mind that reflects upon mantra *becomes* mantra." What does this mean? Basically it is a statement about the nature of the mind. It is also a statement about the nature of the Self, both in its vital power and in its essential capacity to manifest. It means, essentially, that the essence of the mind is nothing but the vibration of the creative energy of Life Itself.

This we experience, at one level, as the extension and contraction of the mind. As a pulsation, the mind is always reaching out for something, bringing it back to absorb and digest, then reaching again and drawing back in. Whenever it reaches out, it gathers up information about the world, reflections on our own existence, activities of other energies, and so on. It does this continually, and on many different levels.

The Zen master Suzuki Roshi described the mind as a swinging door that swings on the breath. It is this pulsation that gives rise to various words, concepts, and images. These, nevertheless, have at the core of their vitality nothing but conscious energy. Moreover, if we put together our understanding of mantra and what the sutra says about the mind, we are led to see that the nature of the mind is nothing but the pulsation of the highest creative energy.

This expansion and contraction of the mind is intimately related to the pulsation of the breath of Life, which is composed of three distinct movements. On one level, it exists as a simple tide that supports our biology. Second, it also exists as a spiral tide, which is our individual inner spirit or energy. Third, it exists as the grand tide which changes our awareness completely. This grand tide has within itself the capacity to reshape and restructure both the spiral tide and the simple tide, and there is a reciprocal relationship between the three.

I use the term tide because if we talk about a pulsation or vibration, we might think of it as something fast, whereas if we talk about a tide, we understand that it happens quite slowly. Nevertheless, this vibration, even though slow, is neither dense nor condensed. It is not like the frequency related to gross matter. Rather it is a free and fluid event.

The mantra practice of the beginning student may start as a prayer — something arising from our sense of ourselves as separate and in need, and as an articulation of our wish for the fulfillment of that need. Eventually, however, we recognize that the fulfillment of the need lies in understanding that our very sense of separateness was like being under the power of a veil whose energies actually have no substantiality at all. Then we know ourselves to be dynamic events.

In the beginning we practice the mantra. In the end the tide of the mantra practices us. We understand that our bodies, minds, and feelings are nothing but the effect of the mantra. In the beginning we think that our effort is the cause and source of the mantra. In the end we understand that mantra is the source of our effort. Then there is no effort. As we move along in our practice and understanding of mantra, we understand these phrases to be the resonance at the very core of our existence. Then the practice of mantra becomes the awareness of the breath of Life pulsating within us. It becomes the tide of the ocean of divine consciousness rising and subsiding within us.

When our self-awareness goes beyond the breathing exercise, it becomes contemplation. More and more our attention turns and is absorbed within, in every activity that we do. Through practice we learn to attune our mind one-pointedly to the vibration of the energy of Life Itself. In other words, the mind becomes completely and intensely attuned to the pulsation of Life Itself.

What is it that gives power to the words we speak? Is it not the love behind them? What is it that gives power to any words at all? The same is true of mantra. It is the feeling from which it springs that is its power. The power of Life Itself — which is love — *that* is the highest mantra of all. When we live from that great reality and let it permeate our understanding, then, because of that love, everything we say becomes a mantra.

The fundamental mantra, or vibration of Life Itself, is really God. At that level no verbalized mantra is needed. We simply attune ourselves to the mantra of Life Itself, which is repeating us. Thus it is not that I *have* a mantra. Rather I *am* a mantra, as is every single person.

To attune the mind totally to that vitality causes us to be identified with it. Because everything is sound and because all sound is simply a manifestation of the energy of Life, then mantra, the person who repeats the mantra, and the goal of the mantra are one. We can never separate the one from the other, because there is no longer any difference between the one who practices the mantra and the mantra itself.

The mind that becomes fully absorbed in that sound becomes that mantra. This takes us into the recognition of the state of Self-awareness. By constant awareness of the real nature of I-consciousness, the mind of the aspirant is transformed into that supreme I-consciousness itself. This is why it is said that the mind that contemplates its own nature *is* mantra.

The whole field of energy — that is, the dynamic expression of energies that we are — becomes attuned to the fundamental vibration of Life Itself. Then it is said in many different texts that every word of the person established in the experience of the Self becomes a mantra, just as every attitude assumed by such a person becomes a mudra, a gesture of the divine.

There is a reciprocal relationship between the highest level of undifferentiated reality and all crystallized form and function. Therefore, mantra is not the enemy of vikalpas; nor is it the destroyer of vikalpas. Rather it is their very foundation. This is why our attunement to mantra ultimately dissolves the appearance of vikalpas. Because we have taken the energy to a deeper level, the tension or crystallization of the first level unwinds.

In the state called nirvikalpa samadhi we are free of all the concepts, thought constructs, and ideas we have about everything. It is not that we have no ideas; nor is it that the mind has no thoughts, feelings, or even any particular personal identity. It simply means that these come and go like waves on the surface of the ocean. Some of them take on a life of their own, move through time and space, and manifest some end. Others have no force at all, and simply melt.

Attunement to that level of vibration leads us to the awareness of a whole range of frequencies operating within us. This is really nothing but the power of the energy Itself, manifesting as us on a moment-by-moment basis. We are nothing but a series of chemistries, or energies, manifesting in a field, and we become aware of that. We recognize the various energies that compel us in different directions for what they are. To see this is to understand the ephemeral nature of our existence. If we can begin to feel the vibrations of all these different chemical events and of the fields of energy that uphold us, we begin to understand the diaphanous nature of our existence.

All of this may sound good and make conceptual sense. I would only add that it is not possible to have a real idea of what I am talking about until one has understood his or her own nature as energy, and developed the capacity to connect deeply to it. This is what allows us to merge our minds into it, to have a genuine communion with it, and to absorb it into ourselves.

When we turn our attention back upon the fundamental nature of our own consciousness and study that — when we turn our awareness back to its source — then the mind that is ordinarily bound becomes the vehicle toward our own freedom. Slowly we begin to recognize the true state of affairs expressing itself in the world: that the mind is an extraordinary vibration, an expression of pure consciousness, a manifestation of brilliance, of conscious light.

The fundamental mantra is God. At that level no verbal mantra is needed. We simply attune ourselves to the mantra of Life Itself, which is repeating us. From the point of view of shaktopaya, mantra is the mind that ruminates over, or participates in, its highest nature and essence.

UNMESHA: THE STILLPOINT

At the moment when one has perception or knowledge of two objects or ideas, one should simultaneously banish both perceptions or ideas and, apprehending the gap or interval between the two, should mentally adhere to it. In that interval will Reality flash forth suddenly.

— THE VIJNANABHAIRAVA

The entire universe is nothing but the opening out, or expansion, of the creative energy. This opening out is called *unmesha*. When the universe draws back into itself, that is called *nimesha*. Together they constitute the essential pulsation of spanda. We talk about them as though they happened one after another, but actually they occur simultaneously. This is because any sequence of events happens in time, and the highest reality is beyond time. So unmesha and nimesha are simply two expressions of the divine. What is unmesha from one point of view is, from another point of view, nimesha. They are not two opposing principles.

Within us, unmesha is the unfoldment of our spiritual awareness. It refers to the opening out, or the disclosing, of the true nature of the Self. It is in the background of all our other thoughts, or vikalpas, but is usually drowned out by all their useless chatter.

The *Vijnanabhairava*, the earliest known foundation text of Kashmir Shaivism, suggests that when we sit in meditation we pay attention to the pause at the end of the inbreath and the pause at the end of the outbreath. These are known as stillpoints. They are the moments in which a shift occurs. The Trika thinkers referred to such moments as *shunya*, or void.

This is not the same kind of void as the Buddhists talk about, although it is related. The main difference is that the Buddhists describe this void as empty, while the Trika masters said that it was an infinitely full and pure potentiality. It is in such a moment that we have direct experience of the dynamic stillness of Life Itself.

We encounter this void at any junction point between two similar energies. For example, it occurs in the stillpoint between two thoughts. When we are involved in one thought and another one comes to us, there is a pause between the two. Unmesha is the disclosure of the true nature of the Self that underlies all the thoughts. At the same time, the void itself is free of all thoughts and can emerge in that stillpoint.

It is not enough to have an intellectual grasp of this void. It can only be experienced in our bodies, breath, and thought. We meet it when we train ourselves to be aware of the stillpoints between our breaths and between our thoughts. This comes about by what is referred to as an alert passivity. Eventually there arises a state in which we are so deeply absorbed in the nature of the stillpoint, the precise point of equilibrium between the breaths and thoughts, that even our awareness of individual breaths or individual thoughts dissolves into that.

This center, or point of equilibrium, that we enter is known as the heart. This is the void that separates all things. It is the intermediate state between them. When we can learn to go from one such point to another as the dominant moments in our awareness, eventually our focus on the breaths or the thoughts surrounding them drops away. What we are left with is a sustained awareness of the true center.

The experience is something like this: Look around you until some object catches your attention. Look at it carefully for a few moments. Then take your attention away from it and direct it into the area of your heart. Focus it there for a while. Notice how, as you direct your attention into your heart, you feel a sense of opening begin to happen.

Staying with that sense of openness, once again look at the object. Notice how your awareness of it has changed as a result of reorienting your attention. Nothing has really moved but the pendulum of your awareness. In taking your attention inside it is not that you became unaware of the object; when you looked at it again you were able to do so with a deeper sense of it. This exercise suggests something of how, when we can learn to sustain the awareness of the heart regardless of what we are looking at or interacting with, we enter into the awareness of the true center.

The paradox here is that we quiet the mind by focusing it on one thing. This takes it beyond its usual tendency to be scattered among many. At the same time, however, what we focus it on is a void. We release ourselves from thinking of anything in particular, and yet we remain intensely aware. So by opening our hearts to the void, we find that what is ordinarily a fleeting moment becomes the central point in which we reside. Then all our experience becomes an expression of what we encounter there.

Therefore, we start out with a specific practice requiring concentration and effort: We train our awareness to focus on the pause between the breaths and our thoughts. This is part of anavopaya. As it unfolds into a different order of awareness, however, the emphasis shifts from effort and technique to awareness of the energy. Thus it emerges into shaktopaya.

The opening out of awareness that we experience is unmesha. Here unmesha literally means the opening of the eyelid, or the uncovering of an essential reality. This has nothing to do with any expression in the world. Rather it is the unfoldment of an inner experience, in which our restlessness and worry are split open. In that gap we encounter a wondrous sweetness and become absorbed in an extraordinary sense of delight.

Abhinavagupta describes this experience as the rupture in two modes of time, the past and the future. We are so absorbed in this sustained present of the center that past and future become irrelevant. Ordinarily our sense of the present depends on there being a past and a future; when these drop away, so does our awareness of "present" as a temporal mode. So we rise above any sense of time at all and become aware, instead, of the infinite energy of Life Itself.

The Trika masters asserted that the individual human being is a microcosm of the cosmos. When they talked about the center, or the heart, they were referring not only to the space of the heart but to the heavens as well. "Heart," in this context, means both the light of consciousness and the basis of the whole universe. It is both the essential Self and the center of all manifestation.

Nityananda talked about it as *chidakash*. *Chit* means "consciousness," and *akasha* means "space," or "sky." So chidakash means "the sky of consciousness." This is synonymous with another term he frequently used — *hrydayakasha*, or "the sky of the heart." This image was central to his teaching.

The energy of the heart is sometimes described as secret or mysterious because we so often remain unaware of it. It is as if we walked around all the time with a secret we used to know but have forgotten. Yet it is present to us all the time. Its infinite sweetness underlies every moment of our lives whether we are aware of it or not. Nor is it really secret, since once we turn our attention to it, it reveals itself.

It is like a seed that has not yet begun to unfold. Its whole reality is present within it, just as a redwood tree dwells implicit within its own seed. In the same way, the entire universe is contained in the center of the heart. This is why Nityananda always urged his devotees to look inward for the truth. He spoke of the royal road to liberation as being within, and often said that the best place to go on a pilgrimage is in the heart. When you see the sunrise in the sky of the heart, he said, it is possible to describe it. But you must see it in yourself.

Nor is it enough simply to enter into the heart as a passing experience. The well-being we experience there is something we sustain only by being steady and vigilant in quieting our minds and emotions, even when we are under great pressure. When we can do this, however, we see that this center, like a deep and quiet pool of water, reflects everything else in its original harmony.

I said earlier that the Buddhists consider the void to be an infinite emptiness. In Trika Yoga thinking, however, it is from a void that the absolute manifests. It is therefore replete with the dynamic vitality of all creation. This is why we say that the energy of the void is the energy of Life Itself. It is a point of infinite possibility.

From the point of view of our practice, therefore, we want to penetrate this center and extend its vitality to all our experience. Our aim is to pierce our own misunderstanding and release all differentiation, in order to sustain an undifferentiating awareness. In this way, we develop the art of entering into the spanda that reveals itself at the center.

This expresses itself as an extraordinary wonderment. This vibration of the heart unifies our entire awareness. Like a wave it flows forth from the heart in a spontaneous outpouring. It is the true nature of all inspiration and the true content of the interior life.

EXTENDING THE ENERGY

When the Heart is in a state of contraction the awakened awareness of the individual self is in fact a state of ignorance. But when this contraction ceases to function, then the true nature of the Self shines forth.

— ABHINAVAGUPTA

In the discussion of anavopaya, I talked about the process of extending our creative energy in terms of releasing tensions and allowing that energy to flow in the form of service. The reason we talk about service in connection with anavopaya is that service connotes the idea of going out and giving something. It suggests the idea of one person doing something for another person, even if what we are doing is not an action but simply the release of a tension. What characterizes this as anavopaya is that we are still involved in dualistic thinking: "I" and "you." So in our interactions with the world around us, we think in terms of *our* doing *something* for *someone else*. We tend to think of the relationship between these parts in terms of an exchange of actions, or maybe things.

As our awareness shifts increasingly into focus on the pulsation of spanda, what we mean by extending our creative energy changes in at least three ways. First, we come to understand that the exchange between ourselves and the world is not one of things and actions but of energy. The Trika masters expressed this in their discussion of sacrifice. So, as we will see, in shaktopaya we are talking not about service but about sacrifice.

Second, as our awareness becomes more refined, we are able to interact with the world in increasingly subtle ways. This means that we can bring about change in correspondingly subtle ways. The Trika masters talked about this extension of our energy in terms of *siddhis*, or spiritual powers.

Third, we understand our participation in the flow of the creative energy of Life Itself in new ways. We have a deepened appreciation of its internal logic as it unfolds in its own extraordinary way. We start to appreciate this logic not only as we recognize it in our experience, but as we find it unfolding within us as well. Our work, increasingly, becomes the process of surrendering our finite wills in order to extend ourselves in what I call the logic of love.

SACRIFICE

> *O Lord Bhairava, this consciousness of mine dances, sings, and rejoices greatly, because as soon as it possesses you, the beloved one, the unrivaled sacrifice which is stability, so difficult for others, is accomplished with ease.*

> — ABHINAVAGUPTA

The Levels of Sacrifice

From the perspective of individual effort we talk about extending the flow of our creative energy as service; in the context of shaktopaya we talk about sacrifice. Like service, sacrifice is both an awareness and a way of action, each of which has a reciprocal effect on the other. If service is the extension of our wish to grow, sacrifice is both the outcome and expression of our one-pointed commitment to growing. It is the release of the bonds we once took to constitute our identities as individuals.

Everywhere in the world there is some recognition that growing spiritually involves a sacrifice. Many religious rituals are expressions of this recognition. If we go across the street to a Christian church, for example, we find the tradition of Jesus giving up his short-term, temporal life into the infinite Life.

At some point in time it seems to have occurred to human beings that it was necessary to share in order to maintain the balance of the environment. Whether this came about as a means of settling territorial disputes or because people hoped that in the process of some exchange their prayers would become more powerful, the notion of sharing became sacrifice. In a very real way this act of sacrifice is the original yoga, because yoga literally means union with God. So throughout the ages human beings have recognized sacrifice as the manner by which we attain union with the broader field of life, and establish harmony between ourselves and others. It is the way we harmonize ourselves with nature, with humankind, and with God.

One of the foundations of the spiritual tradition of India is sacrifice. Even now there are thousands of temples where people are continuously offering their prized material possessions and the fruits of their labor into the fire, symbolic of God and, in the highest sense, of Life Itself.

The gods in these temples are accessible. Their images are visible to all the devotees who enter. The whole system of temples and deities is a means of extending participation in this living event and, further, of encouraging people to cultivate the higher qualities within themselves as an outcome of their participation. This notion prevails even in the most popular forms of Hinduism. Although the Brahmin priests are the exclusive mediators and caretakers of the temples, God is accessible to all.

This is a system in which sacrifice is recognized, in one sense, as everyone's obligation. At the same time, it is also everyone's right. One reason why ritual was created was to extend the opportunity for participation in sacrifice throughout the community as a whole. Few people are able to enter completely into the reality of sacrifice as a living experience that transforms them in a radical way. But many people are able to bring incense, flowers, fruit, money, or whatever they have to offer to a temple and, in a simple, less direct way, can experience and participate in the sacrifice and benefit from it. Ritual, at this level, teaches people symbolically. Insofar as people learn through *doing*, it involves them in a process that bypasses a more cognitive approach to a spiritual teaching.

In this context external sacrifice and ritual are the forms by which the individual is prepared for a more subtle phase of inner work. He or she experiences the benefit of contact with the highest, and is thereby expanded. Nevertheless, the point of this contact for such a person is often the hope of some material benefit. For example, many of the earliest sacrificial hymns were requests for sons, cattle, and victory over enemies, and many people still make offerings with the hope of improving their circumstances.

Over time some people began to practice sacrifice as an art in itself and as an attempt to establish their own communion with some higher aspect of life. At some stage they began to concentrate on the process of sacrifice and, with this maturity, understood that the point of it is to establish ourselves in communion with God. Thoughtful and introspective, these people watched the things they did and tried to see deeply into them. They observed the subtlety of their own desires and actions, and understood that the physical act of sacrifice was their vehicle for communion.

Eventually they recognized that the real sacrifice is a purely internal process. They saw that there is no need for any external ritual, no need to offer up a goat, a cow, or a human being. The real offering is the offering of ourselves, which these other things symbolize. Tantrism took the inner meaning of material sacrifice and translated it into an internalized ritual of sacrifice that the practitioner visualized until he or she reached the recognition of the complete identity of sacrificer, sacrifice, and offering. In fact, the emergence of Tantric spiritual practice was really that of an inner sacrifice.

These insights, over time, were refined into spiritual practices such as Trika Yoga. The early practitioners recognized that sacrifice for material benefits is an expression of a limited awareness. They saw that sacrifice simply for love of God and an appreciation of life is an entirely different level of experience. Finally they said that the person who sacrifices from love alone is the one who understands that the very process of sacrifice is its own benefit.

So it was from the sacrifice itself that their contact with God flowed through them. Through sacrifice a sharing took place and a reciprocal balance was established. It was this process of sharing with God that elevated human beings beyond the experience of mundane time and space into an awareness of a whole different dimension, which we call infinity.

The deepest insight of these people was that sacrifice is all that is happening all the time. It is a universal, living event. This is because all of life is really God sacrificing itself continuously: first, sacrificing its unity into the fire in order to give rise to all individuality and differentiation, and then sacrificing that same differentiation back into the oneness. It does this in an endless process of pouring forth from itself without ever in any way being diminished.

We see the identity of sacrifice and God in the ancient roots of language. The Sanskrit word *hutam* meant "something poured out," or offered with joy. The form this took in ancient Greek was *chuton*, and is observable as the proto-Gothic *gudon*. Many scholars believe that a later, shortened form of this word was "God." So, etymologically, God is both the recipient *of* the sacrifice, and that which is poured forth *in* the sacrifice.

This refers to a reality that is something mystical, magical, and difficult to know. But through the purity of our sacrifice and the depth of our devotion, we gain access to this extraordinary and profound mystery.

The Fire of the Sacrifice

Sacrifice involves fire, which is a symbol of transformation. In ancient times the heat and light of fire frightened away the demons of the night and the predators that roamed the forests and jungles. Thus fire afforded protection. It also made it possible for people to purify their food by cooking it. In every way it brought benefit to their lives.

Some of the earliest peoples used fire as the vehicle to carry their material offerings to the level of the divine. It was the fire that burned and transported their offerings to the gods. As their understanding became more sophisticated, they came to think, instead, of an inner fire created by the friction of the mind rubbing against its own resistance, the structures of the ego. This inner fire, when ignited, gave rise to the intense burning of self-reflection, the vehicle by which people were carried from this world into the highest state.

People would describe the experience of setting themselves on fire through their devotion and prayer and by the intensity of their inner work. The word for the burning they experienced was *tapasya*. Tapasya is not just a figurative description. Nor is it an analogy. It is a physical, chemical reality, a demonstration on the material plane of the nature of the creative process.

Trika Yoga is the practice of generating that inner fire into which we sacrifice our minds, emotions, and egos. Through that process of transformation, we stabilize our awareness in the experience of authentic life. For example, in the *Vijnana-bhairava*, an ancient foundation text of Kashmir Shaivism, one of the exercises described has us imagine ourselves being consumed by fire.

This visualization process becomes a reality as the inner fire of kundalini, which we can also call the fire of love, is awakened. This brings about a transformation in our entire systems. Those times when we are mentally, emotionally, and spiritually on fire change the chemistry of our bodies. This is not something we will into being; it just happens. In the context of our own practice, it is the guru who becomes the fire. From that greater fire a tongue of flame is said to extend and symbolically ignite the student. It is the fire of the divine, the primordial fire, that manifests in the form of the guru.

All fire is essentially one. We don't have eighty-five names for it; whether it be the fire on an altar, in a forest, or at the end of a match, it is all still fire. That fire, transmitted from teacher to student, is the fire that consumes the obstacles within the student and establishes him or her within the unity that is both the guru and God. The student enters into the divine fire that is the guru and becomes that same fire through sacrifice, and only through sacrifice.

This fire is painful. There is never a moment when it doesn't hurt, never a time when we don't feel it. It is just a part of what we offer for the opportunity to participate in the divine creativity that is the very essence of God. After all, when we participate in the fundamental rhythm of this process, it dissolves our egos and destroys what is finite within us even as it nourishes us. Digging into our own flesh and slicing ourselves to the bone is not always all that much fun. However, as people dedicated to this field of creative energy it is simply the price we pay.

In my view, life manages to kick the hell out of all of us in one way or another. So we might as well pay the additional twenty-five percent and go all the way. Real sacrifice is a matter of trading in rocks for diamonds. It is giving rabbit pellets for pieces of gold. What, then, is really consumed in the fire?

Fire is transformation. It breaks down our chemical patterns and crystallizations. It is like what happens in the sun, which makes life possible on earth. The fire of our inner work is what breaks down individualized structures of any kind, and returns their energy into a greater atmosphere. It is the transformation of the individual into the divine. When we can open ourselves to it, we enter into the real depth of all sacrifice and participate in the essence of true communion.

The Offering

We say that sacrifice corresponds to the awareness called shaktopaya because in this phase of awareness, we experience the energy of Life Itself as simultaneously individualized and yet not individual at all. We move on a continuum: Even though we operate as individualized events, we no longer identify exclusively as "I" or "me," because the awakening of the inner fire begins to dissolve these boundaries. We are increasingly aware of something deeper out of which we come.

As this happens, all that isolates us as individuals — our minds, ideas, and desires — begins to be released. In that state we no longer struggle with tensions or with bringing about an opening and flow. Instead, a certain openness naturally comes about and consumes these tensions. We don't see its fire burning; it just happens.

In India the traditional oblation or offering is the butter, sugar, or spice that is poured into the fire. In our own case, however, our individual limitations are what we continuously pour into the inner fire as our sacrifice. This fire is the pure knowledge of our complete, absolute unlimitedness. It is our recognition that all boundaries exist as conventions and conveniences.

A person who recognizes the profoundly ephemeral nature of our bodies and the insubstantiality of this physical, mental, and emotional event understands that, appearances notwithstanding, we are not exactly here as individuals. Our minds and emotions are anything but constant. They change and reorganize themselves moment by moment. So such a person doesn't give all that much importance to these things. Instead, he or she is able to transcend identifying with them. Then a sacrifice has happened: We have given up our bodies and minds to something deeper.

The real sacrifice in our inner work — indeed, the only thing we ever really give up — is the ego. We pour this as the offering into the fire of our quest for truth and our experience of the highest state of pure being. What we are sacrificing is our limited idea of ourselves. Everything we previously identified with the ego we now throw into the fire of our awareness of the Self.

In India this took the form of severing the bonds of caste and one's place in the family. It meant giving up the total identity which, at that time, consisted of the place you lived, the family you belonged to, and the work you did. These people threw all that away. They burned it up and went out into the forests, taking on identities that were far beyond the pale of daily human society. They sacrificed their entire lives and, in so doing, attained an ecstatic state of co-penetration with God.

In our own lives, this same process involves severing our mental and emotional bonds to all the ways we have of establishing our own identities. What does this mean? The *Vijnanabhairava* observes that true adoration consists not in offering flowers and other gifts, but in a deep awareness exempt from dualistic thought.

To transcend the dualism of every feeling and idea is the goal of yoga and of sacrifice. By the discipline of our practice and by selfless participation in the sacrifice, we transcend all the polarities and dualisms: "I'm a good person, I'm not a good person; I am a man, I am a woman; I am this, and not that."

These are means by which we define limited identities. As such they only generate an illusion. This is, first of all, because we rarely see ourselves as we really are. Think, for example, how infrequently we recognize the aspects of ourselves that are truly silly. We are so busy trying to defend some image of ourselves as reasonable, rational, and logical — struggling to sustain some appearance of consistency — that we continuously deny the unreasonable, irrational, and illogical parts of ourselves that never lose power and never evaporate.

This is the identity that consists of all our desires, ambitions, and expectations. It is our entire externalized orientation. The sacrifice of this limited identity is called the unrivaled sacrifice. The work we do to bring this about is an investment we make in ourselves. We weigh the short-term against the long-term interests in our lives. Because we are committed to growing, we sacrifice our short-run comfort, success, and pleasure. In this way it is an investment. At the same time it is a sacrifice that is also an act of worship, a recognition of the absolute value of Life Itself.

What is the connection between growing and sacrifice? Authentic growth, like authentic life, is not located in external experience in and of itself. For example, it is not our jobs or relationships that give authenticity, directness, or real fulfillment to our lives. Just as true love is not the union of two bodies, authentic living is not the accomplishment or acquisition of anything. Rather it occurs when we go beyond the two bodies, beyond any experience of a temporal-spatial order, to participate in the broadest possible range of experience available to us. We sustain our awareness of it even as it coalesces and crystallizes in the form of our everyday lives.

Often what causes us to feel unhappy is that we try to embrace something. Either we end up embracing something dead, or we are unable to embrace that which is truly living. Then, not surprisingly, we feel frustrated. Yet whenever we try to grasp something, it is only the dead things we can get hold of, and never the living. So it is better not to grasp at all. Actually it is impossible. This is why I talk, instead, about participating, or sharing, in an awareness.

When we understand that we own nothing, control nothing, and can hold on to nothing, it becomes possible to sacrifice our boundaries and, especially, our wills. In every sense, what we sacrifice is this small part of ourselves. We do so for the opportunity to experience and participate in a greater part of ourselves. Then we let that greater part go to work as we attain an infinitely expanded sense of identity. Our job is to allow that greatest part of us to function no matter what our individual small minds squawk about as it does so. The process of learning to discriminate between the two becomes clearer as we go.

I was once asked whether the distinction between the individual will and the will of God was a subtle one. I would say that no, the distinction is not subtle. Only when we are entangled in our individual wills does it seem as though it is. The real sacrifice, therefore, is performed from the power of the Self, not of the individual will. It marks our transition into a state of identity with that infinite nature that, as far as the individual is concerned, is one of complete surrender. In that state of surrender, agency is not an issue: All is the elaboration of spirit.

Growing is really the process by which our awareness extends itself through the artificial barriers of time and space — through the insubstantial walls of our minds and emotions — into the essential reality of which we are composed and from which we express ourselves every day. Growing is both a breath that we take and a life that we live. It is the process by which our hearts and minds are elevated beyond the dirt path that most people travel. It is the foundation of beauty. It is what brings stability into our lives because, not desiring anything in particular, we are no longer dominated by desire at any point.

Spiritual Cannibalism

Traditionally the sacrifice we make to bring this about has been described as the food that is offered up. The final sutra in the shaktopaya section of the *Shiva Sutras* says, "*jnanamannam*," or "knowledge is food." It suggests that the limited knowledge that is the cause of bondage is the food to be devoured. These *Sutras* go on to say that "The body becomes an oblation to be poured into the fire of highest consciousness."

Another term for limited knowledge is tension. This tension is food to be consumed by the person established in the awareness of shaktopaya. What we burn up is our tension and resistance, our desires and images — the forms we mold. Limited knowledge is crystallized energy, so it must be consumed and digested. This process of consuming and digesting releases the energy contained within the event, as when anything is burned.

When Rudi talked about "spiritual cannibalism," he used the phrase to represent and make personal the dynamic, chaotic, and powerful process of Life Itself whereby everyone and everything lives upon and from every other. He was describing the process by which Life continuously consumes itself from the simplest to the most sophisticated organisms. One could say that we participate in a total universe, even a total orgy, of consumption. One thing consumes the other, which consumes another, which consumes yet another, and so on. Yet spiritual cannibalism is also the recognition that, while we must eat to live and to grow, we also have a profound responsibility for putting something back into our environment, thereby establishing (or at least maintaining) a dynamic balance. It is within that dynamic balance that the highest state of Self-awareness becomes apparent.

If *jnanam* is interpreted as limited or ordinary knowledge, then the sutra would suggest that limited knowledge is devoured by the yogi. If jnanam is interpreted as knowledge of the Self, then *jnana* would mean the food that gives satisfaction. The whole sutra would then mean that Self-realization becomes a person's food, filling him or her with the highest satisfaction.

The transcendence of tension is, implicitly, the act of self-sacrifice. The tension and burning we feel are this sacrifice while it is still in progress. Its completion brings us to the point of no further fire or tension because there is nothing left to burn.

It is through this sacrifice that we transcend the temporal and spatial structures of our individuated awareness and become established in that state beyond time and space that we would identify as authentic life. Although it uses the structures of time and space to express its creative capacity, true life is never limited by its vehicle, just as an artist is never limited by his or her media but simply uses them to articulate a body of inner feelings.

This experience is one of love going into love, wisdom into wisdom, and understanding into understanding. It is what gives rise to a geometric progression within our practice that establishes us on the shores of creation.

Giving and Receiving

It was recognized long ago that the degree of purity with which a person enters into the sacrifice plays a profound role in the benefit he or she derives from it. People who go into it with some objective in mind are limited in terms of their participation in the effects of sacrifice, as well as in the benefit that can extend through them to the larger community of which they are a part.

A person who understands the essential importance of sacrifice is one whose potential for growth is unlimited. A person who does not sacrifice cannot grow. This is not because God is greedy and demands a ten percent cut of the action but because two things cannot occupy the same space at the same time. If we want to grow, we must create space for change.

By sacrificing we remove a piece of the crystallization that we are and allow for a reordering of all the different parts of ourselves. This happens through the input of a finer energy, which always moves to fill the void. It thereby creates a change in the vibration that we are, restructuring all the remaining components in a higher way.

In being called upon to make some sacrifice in our lives, it is only because of our fear, anxiety, greed, selfishness, stupidity, and misunderstanding that we release something and then immediately fill the void with tension. This only causes the old patterns to reorganize into a denser, or at least similar, frequency. However, when we are able to give with love and purity whatever our lives call upon us to give, it is natural that a finer frequency will manifest within the void that we create by what we have allowed to go.

Here we have the supreme justification for what we can call non-attachment. It is even more than a justification; it is the understanding of non-attachment. We then begin to understand that the highest state continuously sacrifices itself. It sacrifices its own unlimitedness, its absolute peace and repose, in order to breathe life into the spectrum of conscious beings.

It takes something to get something. Nothing is free. Giving and receiving are, together, a mutually balanced process, such that we must always give something if we are to get anything. This is not just a law of economy; it is what structures the process of Life Itself. Exchange is the essence of all relationship, and relationship is the essence of creation.

If we are out to get something out of life, we will always lose. This is the basic rule of what I call the game of life. But if we turn this around and live our lives to give something, then we are no longer playing the game of life in which winning and losing count for everything. Instead, we are living the life of sacrifice.

We could also call this sacrifice a gift because, as a sacrifice, it is freely given and never required. Every human being is endowed with the total freedom of the creative energy of Life. The most fundamental thing we value within ourselves and others is this freedom, our right always to choose.

No matter what the political or governmental context, this can never be taken away from us. Only we can give it up. Our sacrifice is never a gift we are compelled to give. Rather it is something we do as part of our decision to experience the awareness implicit in the experience of sacrifice. It is giving our lives away that renews and expands them. It is not the life we have that grows; we give that away and get a bigger one. We give *that* away, and a still bigger one comes. Finally there is no possibility for any more extension because we have become established in the experience of infinite life.

It is not getting we should think about but giving. In the stage of our practice that involves individual effort, we train not to get but to give. In the second phase, it is giving itself that becomes the foundation of our experience of well-being. Because we are giving it all away, what is there to be attached to?

This is equivalent to participating in the universal creative process, which carries us to the point where there is neither giving nor getting. At that point giving and receiving become one thing, and there is only the infinity of the divine presence. It is by the sacrifice of our own limits that we are elevated to an exalted state of awareness. The joy and well-being always present within that highest state manifest as the *prasad*, the gifts of the divine, to those who sacrifice well.

Prasad is a term, in India, that refers to the distribution after the ritual of whatever has been sacrificed. You might, for example, bring some food and offer it. After the sacrifice is made, all this food has been cooked. The priests don't just burn it up; instead, they symbolically offer it up and, afterwards, distribute it to all the people as a symbol of the return on their gift.

This is because the sacrifice is never a one-way street. Giving and receiving are always happening at the same time. The understanding here, however, is that only an ignorant person gives something material and then demands something equivalent in return. There are parables in ancient India about the idiot who brings food to a king and who, when given jewels in return, insults the king because the king has not given him back food. Being a stupid person, the idiot does not recognize the immense value of the jewels or their capacity to buy a hundred thousand times more food than he had offered in the first place. So prasad is not merely the distribution of the benefits of the sacrifice; it implies that something has been multiplied qualitatively.

The real return is love. Anyone who makes the sacrifice purely — with great love and every honest intention, without doubts or the desire for some benefit — slowly comes to understand that, in fact, love is the only sacrifice. Moreover, the sacrificer, the sacrifice, and the recipient of the sacrifice are really one. What binds the one making the offering, the one receiving it, and the offering itself is one thing, and that is always love.

In a way, authentic love is always a kind of sacrifice that happens from an awareness of universal integration and unity. It is not the love we usually think of as occurring between two people. We could also put it this way: Jesus once said, "No greater love has a person than to lay down one's life for a friend."

Paradoxically, a person who attains the highest state has no reason or personal need to be particularly interested in the existence of any other. Yet, repeatedly, such a person chooses to relate to others, to extend him- or herself into the world to deal with pain and suffering, and to do and give without any concern for what he or she is getting out of the whole thing.

What this requires is giving of ourselves. We are not doing so for the sake of any other person; rather we are sacrificing ourselves into the Self. In another words, we are sacrificing the small self in order to realize the great Self. Every time the small self dies, it is like the death of a weed. It allows our highest Self to have more space in which to rise up and flourish.

As I am talking about it, love and God are the same thing. Love is the conscious capacity to give endlessly of ourselves, without ever experiencing any depletion. It is the capacity to live from and express our connection to the infinite resource. The sacrifice of love into love only gives rise to more love. From this, a universal awareness emerges.

Into All Realms of Our Lives

When we talk about extending our creative energy, how does this pertain to sacrifice? The yogis, long-haired ascetics, and other early spiritual types were intent on extending the sacrificial ground into the whole material world and in turning their entire lives into a sacrifice. For them the sacrificial ground became wherever they went, and as far as they could see or imagine. The sacrificial fire was their own life force. Its fuel was their bodies; the offering, their senses, minds, and emotions. It was this sacrifice that brought them into contact with the divine.

Extending the energy and extending the sacrifice were, for them, one and the same thing. It meant that there was nothing outside the realm of the sacrifice. Everything well done was considered a part of it, and further, an expression of some higher creative energy bringing blessing into a person's life.

This is no less true of every arena in our experience. Think of your work in the world, for example, as simply setting the stage for this sacrifice. Each activity is one of the things you do to prepare for it. Together they constitute the clearing of the space, the preparation of ritual objects, the gathering of special flowers. More importantly, the ultimate point of all this preparation is to cast everything into the fire: not to cherish anything for itself but to give everything away and release it all. The great Sufi teacher Rumi says:

> *The sufi opens his hands to the universe*
> *and gives away each instant, free.*
> *Unlike someone who begs on the street for money to survive,*
> *a dervish begs to give you his life.*

So we engage in our work in the world not out of a compulsion to attain something from it but out of generosity. That way we don't skimp on the flowers or buy cheap wine for the offering. Because we have value, we bring value.

For that matter, we do not do our work to acquire something we don't have but to demonstrate something we already *do* have and always have had. In order to do this we must also be people who are thoroughly educated and capable of going into a brutally secular world without being disturbed, unbalanced, or left unable to function by it. If our sacrifice is effective, it must be so throughout all the realms of our lives and not just one alone.

When we talk about mixing our spiritual practice and our material, ordinary world, we are also saying that it is a sacrifice. The whole process of any ritual, which is the material manifestation of sacrifice, involves bringing that highest essence down into ordinary life. It is a mixing, a process by which we transform time and space, earth, water, fire, and air, into something sacred. We reduce all those material manifestations to their most primordial nature.

In that way we have not extended the actual sphere of the divine; rather we have extended our recognition of that sphere. We have recognized that all the elements that are the very components of our material existence and our everyday lives are nothing themselves but expressions of the divine. As we see in every act a ritual of sacrifice, we recognize the world as one with God. Through this process — through our practice, through extending ourselves in service, and through giving — we express our participation in this extraordinary communion.

Our concern is to live in that state. In the same way that early human beings recognized the intrinsic benefits of sacrifice, there is likewise for us a benefit that automatically extends itself through the process of our sacrifice to the whole of humanity. It is not that we do anything as a favor to anyone else; what we do springs simply from our recognition that it is necessary in our own lives.

All human beings benefit from this sacrifice in which we burn up our limited lives. This is a form of service. In a very real way, anything we do to refine the environment by lifting ourselves out of our own tensions is an improvement. If one person is happy no matter what is going on around him or her, this can only advance the general condition of the total environment.

Furthermore, if one person can take on and burn off the tensions of those around him or her, this opens up the field of possibility even further for all involved. Think, for example, of all the bodhisattvas in the Buddhist mythology. They no longer have any personal self-interest, but refrain from passing over into nirvana in order to further the process of awakening among all sentient beings. Their lives are a constant self-sacrifice for the benefit of the world.

The service that we discussed as part of our practice in anavopaya is, in a very real way, the sacrifice we undertake. It is the arena in which we make our offering on a daily basis by physically grounding that state of total well-being in this world. It is the way we take this sacred space, which is the state of God, and bring it directly into our own lives.

This makes it possible for all human beings, in one way or another, to participate in the ongoing divine process of sacrifice. We do so for the benefit of all those whose lives we touch, and for the benefit and stability of the greater environment. The consideration and kindness we show to every other, whether these be the people we care about or those we don't, is service. Our real sadhana begins with commitment and ends as service. The event, as a whole, is sacrifice.

Conclusion

We may not accomplish the sacrifice without first making the essence of the energy our own. We can easily buy the substances that serve in ordinary worship, but nowhere at any price can we purchase the true offering. This is our deepest awareness of the Self. True worship happens when we become conscious that our own nature is identical with this highest reality. In this process the adorer and the adored become one.

When we understand that consciousness contains everything in itself, then any activity becomes a rite of devotion. Therefore, why should we go to worship God in a church or a temple when our own bodies are tabernacles and our own awareness and energy the divinities to receive our love and devotion?

When we know this, our lives in the world become simple. We may or may not have the trappings of worldly success, but we do have an inner fullness, a sense of maturity and joy within ourselves that transcends the ephemeral nature of our experience and goes beyond all financial success and worldly recognition.

This richness within ourselves we cannot lose. If we give it away, it comes back twofold. This is a win-win proposition. It is the classic double-bind in reverse. We cannot lose. Then we live our everyday lives doing whatever we need to do to support this atmosphere of lightness and warmth around us.

This does not mean we become flaky. It means we live with discipline and simplicity in order not to create tension. When we do face tensions we deal with them straightforwardly, looking to see what our responsibility is and how it might be carried out in a manner beneficial to all concerned.

Then the happiness we feel within ourselves becomes something we extend to other people. We don't do things that will not promote happiness among others — not because we are particularly altruistic, but because that is what we have to do to promote happiness in our own lives. So what we end up with is a win-win situation between ourselves and others as well.

The more we carefully examine the universal process of sacrifice, the more we recognize the extraordinary infinity in which we participate and which we are. This is what dissolves our boundaries, limitations, and every distinction. At the same time, in our everyday lives it brings us complete peace because we have the experience that we are complete and whole.

This allows us to dwell in peace as we are. We don't concern ourselves about coming or going, gaining or losing. We live in constant awareness of the profound uncertainty that this infinity is. This uncertainty no longer terrifies us, because we experience it as something joyous and full of infinite possibility.

Through this understanding, our torn lives are unified. Each aspect of our lives becomes woven into the fabric of every other aspect of our lives. There is a wholeness on every level that brings a great ease and comfort, a graciousness that is present no matter what kind of stress and strain overtake us. It is sacrifice that essentially establishes our place in the cosmos and maintains the harmony of that place. It is what gives us access to the experience of the whole.

Sacrifice is the essence of spirituality. It is the process by which, as individual human beings, we are reunited with our essential nature. The core experience that brings this about is our awareness of the energy, the simple fluctuation of the divine, vital breath. This is our awareness of spanda, which comes to us the more we release our boundaries.

Again, surrender is really the issue here. There *is* no other issue. A person who participates in this sacrifice gains a depth and confidence in surrender and is ultimately able to let go of attachment to everything. Surrender permeates the notion of sacrifice. Ultimately the unrivaled sacrifice *is* surrender. So whenever we talk about surrender, we are also talking about the act and process of sacrifice.

At the deepest level of the sacrifice there is only surrender. There is no individual and nothing related to the individual to talk about. Even as we move about in our individual lives after that, we cannot imagine that we are *doing* anything. Rather the point is that God can do anything at any time, and does. We ourselves are only one expression of that creative energy.

SIDDHIS: THE POWER OF THE ENERGY

You are lucky if you work for years without any sign of the miraculous. You are building a strong mechanism. You might envy those who see or hear "the spirits." Don't — these lesser gifts are to be cast aside so that greater forces can work for you.

— RUDI

The Power Trap

Most of us enter the spiritual search quietly looking, in one way or another, for the power to fulfill some desire or exercise greater control over our own lives. We want the power to use our words and actions to attain success and recognition in the world, to get something out of life. More basically, we experience a lack of creative flow on one level or other in our field of existence. Sensing that our lives are not what they could be, we undertake some sort of spiritual practice.

There is nothing wrong with such reasons for entering a spiritual life. Nor is there anything wrong with the initial changes we hope to bring about. In themselves these are good things. If we draw them out to their logical conclusion, however, they ultimately become nothing more than the quest for power. This, in turn, can deteriorate into spiritual materialism, the worst form of materialism imaginable. It is greedier, more lustful, and more corrupting than any other form of materialism because it is all the more subtle.

In texts such as the *Shiva Sutras*, we find references to unusual capabilities that manifest in a person who pursues liberation. These powers have a certain vague status because they are, in a way, supernatural, even as they also function in the world of limited time and space. In the classical system they are known as the *ashtanga siddhis*, the "eight powers," or simply, *siddhis* ("powers").

Siddhis, or unusual capabilities, are likely to arise within a person who has fulfilled the awareness of shaktopaya. Many of these capabilities coincide with the ability to participate in increasingly subtle levels of vibration. That being the case, in varying degrees a person becomes able to reorganize experience itself. That is, since there is but one conscious energy that unfolds as the entire range of inner and outer experience, it is possible for us to learn to alter the structure of our experience on an extremely refined level.

In one sense siddhis are a natural outcome of our practice and of the refinement of our awareness. Yet the *Shiva Sutras* also state emphatically and repeatedly that to engage in them reflects an immature state of spiritual realization. Thus, they are the manifestation of ignorance and confusion. To get involved in demonstrating such powers only further draws a veil over the highest reality.

Most importantly, they are not proper or appropriate to the long-term development of our real creative ability. Consequently, they themselves become a source of additional confusion. They are the outcome of our delusion about the essential nature of the Self, and by such means, we cannot realize the highest reality.

We see demonstrations of people with siddhis in many settings. Anybody who is profoundly sincere in any religious tradition, or who has true commitment, cannot help but experience real inner power and the capacity to communicate that power to others. This does not necessarily mean the person has the slightest understanding of what he or she is doing. It is all too easy for the ego to get involved and to get lost in greed, power, and lust. Furthermore, once a person starts to manipulate others, guilt and internal conflict also come into the picture.

It is undeniable that the most important element in the development of any spiritual power is a person's total commitment. Not surprisingly, however, *what* we are committed to has a profound effect on our awareness and shapes the nature of the outcome of our work. Look, for example, at the late Ayatollah Khomeini of Iran. He was totally committed to the destruction of the Shah and to vengeance. He developed enormous powers of hatred and, in the process, used them not to create life but to destroy it.

I do not find the case of the Ayatollah admirable, but in the big picture, he is an example of enormous power. Real commitment to anything manifests as power. Anybody with a total commitment to something can manifest it; such power is open to anybody. The good and the righteous don't have a lock on siddhis. I do not acknowledge this lightly, but it is true.

At the same time, the nature of our commitment will also be the limit of what we are able to attain. The power it brings about, in and of itself, is not automatically synonymous with well-being, peace of mind, or growth. I said earlier that any total commitment ultimately leads to love, but that happens only when a person is authentically committed to growing as a human being. Otherwise, ambition goes to ambition, and hatred to hatred. This is so even when it bears the label of some high-sounding religious or political ideal.

The distinction is that a total commitment to growing, to universal integration, and to total well-being is also a total commitment to encompassing and transcending all power. It is a commitment not only to immerse ourselves in the state from which power emerges in the first place; it is also a resolve to reside there without being tainted by that power and without buying into the limitations implicit in any human endeavor. Then we are able simply to serve whatever situation we find ourselves in.

The emergence of siddhis is a tricky event because it is so easy to get the wrong idea about what is going on, thereby reentering a condition of delusion. The risk in terms of authentic spiritual work arises when we pay attention to power, identify with it, and get involved in it. Then our emotions, desires, fears, ambitions, and needs all fuse into tension and struggle that obscure the pure, remarkable capabilities implicit in the real power of Life Itself.

Interest in siddhis is just another form of acquisitiveness and greed. The problem with this inferior capacity is that it still represents an attachment to the arc of material existence. Like this arc, it arises and subsides. To engage in such powers on a personal level for some personal reason is to demonstrate a purpose, even if it is ostensibly a spiritual purpose. This intent once again sets in motion the externalization of our attention and the need for some sense of accomplishment. From there we are back into the cycle of ambition, gain, and loss.

Anyone who achieves a certain level of awareness in his or her work has to be careful about becoming impressed by his or her own capability. The minute our minds get involved at any level, we tend to take credit in one way or another for what is going on. We end up with a problem on our hands because we identify ourselves as some kind of hotshot. Then it is adios, mother.

Rudi used to tell a story about a Tibetan monk who was highly gifted. Every morning at four o'clock all the monks in the monastery sat in meditation. One night, this particular monk experienced levitation. He became so excited by this that instead of walking into the meditation hall the next morning, he floated in over the other monks. They were all extremely impressed. But, said Rudi, six months later this same monk was working in a circus.

Getting caught up in these kinds of things is ultimately a no-win situation. If we are working within ourselves to bring about a change and it somehow happens, the next thing we know we are thinking, "By God, I'll bet there are a lot of other changes I can make happen and, son of a gun, maybe I can even figure a way to make a buck out of it." We become acquisitive, and the next thing we know we have become what Rudi used to call magicians. He observed that the material life around such people may increase, but others whose lives they touch do not become free.

When we become acquisitive, we start to identify in subtle ways with the idea that we are *getting* something out of our spiritual work. Eventually that acquisitiveness becomes a real source of constipation, because we end up taking inventory of what we have and of our own capability. Then we get caught up in feeling that people are not recognizing who we are or what we deserve and that our entire contribution has gone unnoticed. This, to put it bluntly, is a bucket of crap.

Nityananda used to say that the three K's were the obstructions to our inner work. These were *kanaka* ("gold" or "greed"), *kanta* ("lust"), and *kirti* "the desire for name and fame". He used to say that these obstructions occurred in ascending order, becoming more subtle and difficult to overcome. Many, he said, would overcome the first two, only to be overset by the thirst for recognition and fame. The problem is that any power that generates an attachment to actions and their results is an obstacle to our freedom.

This includes discovering that our capacity extends to siddhis of a psychic nature. If this happens, we may think we can know what is going to happen in the future. Maybe it even turns out that we *do* know a few times. Then we go on to try and use this ability, in which case we either become an entertainer or we turn it into a business and stop doing our real work. Then we find that even though we may be right for a while, we are just as often wrong. We start thinking, "What's wrong with me? What happened?" All of this creates more confusion and problems than it ever resolves.

Power is an enormous trap. Once we get locked into some purpose, however noble, it is not long before that purpose takes over and leads us into politics. From there it becomes a prison. We spend our power, exhausting both it and ourselves in the process, at which point we are finished. It is a rare person who can be a vehicle through whom power flows without being tainted by the power itself. That is the constant challenge, and one that requires constant vigilance.

The Delusion of Helping Others

Many people begin with a sincere commitment, develop a certain level of power, and fall. They become entangled in and consumed by the power they have attained, and because of having engaged their ambition and attempted to use these powers, they are reduced to an even lower level than before. This has been my observation, as well as something warned against by various foundation texts of the tradition.

The reason for this is simple. To demonstrate greed in the field of highly intense energy will intensify that greed tremendously and bring a person quickly to a low level within him- or herself. The experience may initially seem interesting or exciting, but from a spiritual point of view it is not nourishing in the slightest. There had better come a point where we recognize this, because if we don't, we will be sinking like a stone along with every dream we have ever known. Unless we have a real commitment to a deeper understanding that supercedes any kind of entanglement, we are going to go down with it when it goes down.

This may not be a fundamentally important distinction in the beginning, but as we go along and as things start to change, we cannot afford to be satisfied with the development of the limited powers that emerge from the experience of the inner Self. Indeed, we must be always alert to every kind of nonsense that asserts itself, certain that it will all pass by us if we are determined to grow.

It says in the *Shiva Sutras* that a fully enlightened person must remain vigilant at all times lest he or she get entangled in the various levels of activity that ensnare other people. In other words, having the highest understanding, or even a flash of great insight into the nature of Life Itself (and there is no human being who has not), is no guarantee against forgetting about doing our inner work.

Our minds are like plugs. We plug them into whatever power source we want, represented by what we desire, by the goals we set, and by the nature of our ambition. We could almost say that our ambition represents a voltage. When we plug our minds into it, that is the power that will flow through and from us. When we plug our minds into the highest, however, what flows through us is the power of the highest. It has nothing to do with ordinary ambition, because we identify only with that highest, and with nothing else.

Our relationship to our experience involves our relationship to what we identify as ourselves. As this identity becomes increasingly clear, our relationship to our experience changes. In the process the appropriateness of our ambition becomes suspect. Slowly we understand that authentic ambition has nothing to do with our success or failure. Rather it has to do with recognizing the emptiness of the rewards for all human endeavor. This recognition generates the motivation that compels us to know the essence of all endeavor. When we know this, what attraction can limited powers hold for us?

Of course, we may think we are engaging in such expressions of power in order to benefit others, which should make it all right. Are we not, after all, aiming to serve them? Yes, but not in this way. To think that we can is still a delusion. Who, after all, are we really helping? Of the things I have seen that pass for benefit to other human beings, 99.9 percent of them are nothing of the kind.

In fact, the minute we insist we are going to do something for somebody else, we have just put our head in the toilet. That other people perhaps experience benefit from something we do is a wonderful thing, but once we decide that *we* did it, we have just sent ourselves right back onto the down escalator. Rudi used to put it even more bluntly. He thought that anyone who feels a need to "help the world" or who is operating on any other kind of large-scale visionary ideal is a fool.

To attempt to help somebody else because we think he or she needs an act of our compassion is the same as seeking some kind of self-aggrandizement. Thus, at various points we have to examine our motivation. The acquisition of powers and the assumption that, in some way, we can do good with them, is no more legitimate than the acquisition of a doctrine and the notion that we can be missionaries and do good with *that*. Whoever needs help will ask for it, at which point we can give it simply.

As long as we are dealing with symptoms and problems, as long as we are trying to fix somebody, we are basically monkeying with something we don't understand. Then, generally speaking, it bites us. A person who attains the highest state and is stabilized therein is open like the sky at night and giving like the sun. The presence, warmth, fullness, and joy implicit in this connection to the highest state gives all. It just is. The sun does not have the idea that its powers operate for the benefit of anybody. It is just there, doing what it does. It so happens that doing what it does makes it possible for us to exist. So we are grateful.

Real Power is Not Dramatic

Different collections of miracle stories (or what I think of as the spiritual comic books) sometimes emphasize siddhis in such a way that they can appear to be one of the objectives of spiritual work. When we read or hear about these powers, we may either dismiss them as accounts of the deluded faithful or we may buy into them as significant proof of inner accomplishment. Yet I would suggest that between cynicism and gullibility there lies a third way of understanding such powers.

It is true that there are people who can do startling things. I have been to India many times and have seen several people there who have the ability to manifest objects. One of them has hundreds of thousands of people come to see him. He gives them ashes and candy, or sometimes watches, jewels, and other such things. I have seen him do this three or four times and have received things from him myself. It is pretty remarkable to see his hand turn blue and then have all kinds of hardware fall out of it. It looks as though he has the other hand stuck into some kind of astral pawnshop.

There are many different kinds of miracles. I once met a man in India who sits under a tree holding on to a sock. All day long he pulls fruit out of it, and a lot of people come to see him do it. He gives people bananas, apples, and other fruit. Furthermore, he doesn't put anything into the sock ahead of time. I myself don't know how he does it, nor do I particularly care.

These are the kinds of activities that impress people, although they are less impressive after you have been around them for a while. It means that we have to read stories of the lives of saints not with cynicism but with understanding of the human tendency to characterize the appearance of such situations improperly.

I say this because if somebody says to you, "This incredible miracle happened in my life. Swami So-and-So did this, and somebody else did that," then what happens? You may start to think, "How come that hasn't happened to me?" The whole thought invariably loops around to some version of "What's wrong with me? Why am I not getting this?" Then we become either jealous and depressed, or in some way insecure. This is a tremendous waste of time.

The danger of collecting miracle stories about anybody is that these become the wrong focus of our attention. In fact, not one of these stories is really the substance of anyone's existence. Rudi, in fact, continuously denounced the whole interest. He felt it was, and is, nothing but another form of spiritual materialism.

The nature of the miraculous is such that it does little to connect a person more deeply with him- or herself. Moreover, these powers don't really help anybody. One example is the different kinds of visions a person might have in meditation; another is the variety of psychic or clairvoyant experiences. Different things can happen spontaneously, such as having beautiful fragrances surround us in meditation. All of this is pretty much a case of glitz. When we take it seriously, then it is more on the order of a delusion and is counterproductive to our inner work.

I would have to say that I have never seen a person who has really grown spiritually as a result of such experiences. I have never seen anyone who became stronger within him- or herself or who cultivated a deeper contact with the highest reality within him- or herself as a result. This is because there is a tendency to get hooked on miracles and become attached to external phenomena. This is not entirely surprising. After all, these spectacles are fascinating. Nevertheless, this does not make them important.

If we are looking for drama, we are going to miss the real show. To have dramatic experiences may be wonderful in itself, but to become entangled in or dependent on the drama is something totally different. To use it as justification or proof of our growth is a real problem because we become nothing but drama junkies. From there it only gets worse.

Real power is not dramatic. In no way does the reality of the event compare either to the propaganda that we read in the Indian spiritual books or to the drama the Christians make it out to be. Even though the occurrence of miracles is quite real, it is not nearly so flashy as it is presented to be. Any time such information is transferred by word of mouth, we have to factor in people's favorite pastime of exaggeration and one-upsmanship. The characterization, in other words, is inadequate and misses the most important aspects.

Understand that the miracle of Life Itself unfolds in a simple, natural way. This is the main thing. It is not complicated, and none of it is preceded by fanfare. The important experiences are not showy, and no angels descend to kiss us on the nose. We don't sit down and have God whisper in our ear, after which we suddenly put on an incredible performance.

Incredible performances are, first and foremost, the result of long years of tremendous effort. Second, there is no anticipating how the various elements will come together at one particular time in such a way that something extraordinary rolls out of a person. There is no telling how this also happens to be bigger than his or her limited capacity, even though for some reason (we could say, perhaps, because of grace) something truly amazing has indeed happened.

Nityananda spent years in seclusion, wandering from place to place and meeting people only rarely. He could find people when he wished to, but nobody could find him. He didn't receive questions or dispense any teaching. For that matter, we could not characterize anything Nityananda ever did as teaching anybody anything. He never had the intention of doing so. His only intention was to remain in the stability of the highest state, which was all he did and was, in fact, all he was.

For about eight years he lived in a small cave about five feet deep. The cave itself was tucked in a wrinkle of a hillside where nobody else lived, because there were too many snakes, insects, and wild animals. When he finally moved a little ways off the hillside, he found a giant mound of stone down on the other side of the river and next to town. He had people drill through the rock in three straight lines and make two connective tunnels, from which they cut cubicles throughout the whole thing. That was his first ashram.

On one occasion some officials who served the British came and asked him where he was getting all the money for this project. So he took them down to a nearby swamp in which there was every wild thing imaginable. When they got there, he dove in and stayed under water for several minutes. Then he popped up again with two big bags of money in his hands, put them down, and said, "I keep the money down here. Come on, I'll show you." They all ran away and didn't bother him after that. People used to ask him how they were to pay for everything, and he would say, "Oh, the money is under that rock. Just go and get it."

I do not think that anybody can reasonably compare him- or herself to Nityananda or, in fact, to anybody else. Each life has its own extraordinary capability. There is no significant comparison to be made between our inner connections and those of somebody like Nityananda. The only real issue is the degree to which we cultivate our connection ourselves.

We can also make a fundamental distinction between the things we do consciously and the things that happen on their own. When a person makes an attempt to manifest certain kinds of powers, this becomes something he or she *does*. It is different from simply having things happen. For instance, around both Nityananda and Rudi things just happened.

I recall one occasion when another person and I were working in Rudi's art store. Rudi had asked us to move a large Burmese figure of the Buddha into the window. It was a reclining Buddha, about fifteen feet long, five feet wide, and maybe four feet tall. We had to get through a four-foot wide doorway and the angle around which we had to move it was sharp. Not too surprisingly, we were having all kinds of trouble getting the piece to go anywhere.

I was on one end of it when the person pushing the other end said, "Rudi, this will never work" Rudi moved him out of the way and, as he put his hands on the thing, said, "*Never* say never." The next thing I knew, we were right in the window with the Buddha. I have thought about this over and over since it happened. I did not see us move from point A to point B, but we definitely did.

I don't know if Rudi did that or if it just happened, but Rudi ordinarily did not *do* things. He was not impressed by that kind of event, and he made various statements against getting mixed up in them. Still, extraordinary things took place around Rudi that were absolutely unexplainable. Actually, so many of them tended to happen that, in a way, they came to seem almost commonplace. Such things served to reaffirm our basic experience and conviction that we were in a mind-boggling place, but nobody ever talked about them much or seemed to give them any great importance.

The real point is that none of these stories tells us what is most important about either Nityananda or Rudi. The biggest miracles are not the ones that we can see or that capture our minds but the ones that free our minds and promote the unfolding of the simple miracle of Life Itself from within us.

Never to Be Deliberately Exercised
So what should our approach be to these experiences as they come up in our own lives? In our practice there is a

whole process of concentration and meditation on, as well as absorption into, the various levels of awareness. Each of these is represented by different experiences and different practices. We find, in the process, that within the deepest, most personal part of us there also arise all of the capabilities of the universal that can be articulated in the realm of individual existence.

As we become established in the highest level of Self-awareness, the limitations imposed by our biology and its imperatives, by our sensory awareness, and by our contact with the objects of those senses begin to loosen up. I would say that the most important thing for us to understand is that once we penetrate this biological cloud and grasp the fundamental source of our presence here, we also recognize our bodies, minds, and emotions to be only one level of experience in a much broader field of creative activity. As we develop our capacity to stay attuned, and as we become deeply conscious people, a vitality rises from within us. This is simply a finer expression of the power implicit in our gross existence.

By becoming aware of the energy that manifests as the physical body, and by becoming aware of its structure and tuning into that, we find that the whole field of function we call a body changes. Sometimes this is a subtle change, sometimes a dramatic one. Whether subtle or dramatic, however, such change has a powerful impact on the field of experience that manifests as this biological event. As the cloud of our attachment to external objects breaks up and as we have a deeper understanding of our own creative capacity, certain energies manifest within this greater field of highly refined, conscious energy. These energies are unusual and remarkable when seen from the perspective of the ordinary.

Likewise, our awareness of increasingly refined patterns of creative energy and our ability to tune into those energies allows us to generate change within the various fields of our experience. These are sometimes subtle changes that nobody else sees; sometimes they can be quite noticeable. It might happen, for example, that we develop certain capabilities that will manifest themselves spontaneously during the course of our everyday responsibilities. These are like gifts and talents that express themselves naturally and that are both apparent and unapparent at the same time.

The point is simply to allow them to happen, expecting nothing from them and remaining unconcerned about whether they ever happen again or not. As long as we leave the whole thing on this level, the appearance of such events is remarkable, wonderful, and fine. The best thing to do is take it in stride and not even touch it with our minds. Just say, "Thanks a lot," and keep going. It is when we start thinking of ourselves as big shots who deserve something that we kill the goose that lays the golden eggs.

To put it more strongly and explicitly, the powers we experience in this way are never to be deliberately exercised. My agreement with my own teacher was that I would never use spiritual abilities to do anything that could be done in some other, more ordinary way. For example, I was never to contact anyone by extraordinary means as long as it was possible to pick up the telephone. Rudi insisted upon this because any attempt to exercise such powers is a demonstration of greed and gross understanding.

We have every responsibility for the power that emerges through our inner work. It does not make us important. There is a scene in a Japanese samurai movie between the actor Toshiro Mifune and a noblewoman whose life he has just saved. They are sitting in a barn and Mifune is scratching his face. They begin a conversation, and finally she says to him something like this: "You are like a sword out of its scabbard. You gleam too much. The very best swords never leave their scabbards."

People who have real power do not use it. They do not need to. The greatest swordsmen never have to draw their swords. To refrain from using such power saves us from wasting our time and energy and keeps us aware that our real concern lies in learning to participate continuously in a simple state of pure awareness.

The joy that we experience in the vitalization of all levels of our existence is an experience transmitted to all whose lives we touch. The real miracle is the simple, expanded awareness of the power of Life Itself within us. Furthermore, it is the energy that does everything, in every single case. To embrace the notion that *we* are doing anything is to distance ourselves from an awareness of the total unity of all things and to express a proclivity for attachment. When we start believing any hype about ourselves — especially our own — we are worse off than when we began.

Furthermore, the point is not what we are doing but where our attention is. We want to keep everything simple because the truth is that it *is* simple. That is why most of the people who try for it miss it. They are always making it more complicated than it really is. Indeed, our major challenge as students is to not make things more complicated than they are — and they are not complicated. After all, if the highest thing is actually unformed and unmanifest, then it is also the simplest among all the levels of reality.

So our real effort is to make ourselves simple enough to participate in the whole with care and clarity. That is why we don't dope our minds with drugs or our bodies with cigarettes and alcohol. It is why we don't clog our lives with ambition and desire, and why we keep ourselves relatively simple and pure. We work to sustain an environment that allows us to engage in this simple level of the highest reality.

The best thing is to have a long-term point of view, to look to the highest and not be satisfied with anything else. Then if we grow and something remarkable happens around us in the process, we don't even notice it because we are too busy doing our work and going where we are going. With that, it simply becomes one of the features of our unfoldment to that highest state.

It is our love of God and our immersion in the divine that represent a level of flow that does what it needs to do. We are here to serve that flow, not to have any ideas in our minds about what we want to have happen or what we want to accomplish. Having full understanding of that, we enter into the highest consciousness. At that point the creative capacity, the core of what we are, is no longer conditioned by material limitations. None of our ordinary assumptions function in that sphere to limit our attention. This makes the whole continuum of time and space, as well as what lies beyond it, accessible to us.

Be serious about your work and devoted to it. Do it with love, because it is what gives life to your life. But also recognize that your goal is to find not the power but the joy implicit in the highest simplicity. Remember that, and try to find within yourself that simplicity. From your love and devotion try to find a simplicity and lightness that allow you not only to merge into and participate in but also to observe carefully, and slowly to understand this highest and most amazing level of existence.

THE LOGIC OF LOVE

> *When you become aware of the art in a human being, the creative flow in a human being, you really do not need much. There is so much to love, there is so much beauty, there is so much flow, there is so much perfection, there is so much of a wonderful nature to relate to that you do not have to pick at all the small things. It is your bigness that makes everything beautiful.*
>
> — RUDI

The Logic That is Internal

In many of our relationships we get caught up in trying to change the other person. Often, as we saw in the discussion of siddhis, we do this thinking we are really out to help somebody else. However, this is not what is meant by the integration of sacrifice into our lives. Sacrifice is the release of our boundaries. This has nothing to do with imposing our vision, our will, or our power on anybody else.

How, then, does the process of extending ourselves in an authentic way take form in our interaction with others? First and foremost, it involves recognizing and respecting that the energy of Life Itself functions according to an internal logic of its own in every person. The most we can do is try to recognize where it is going. Then we do what we can to let it unfold both in ourselves and in the people around us.

There is a lot we may not understand about this process at any given moment, but when we are centered and established in our own clarity, we don't even have to ask. This logic will reveal *its* intention and *its* power. As this happens, we come to recognize that relationships are self-revealing phenomena: Through our simple participation in them, they disclose what they are. If we put too much energy into them, we simply unbalance them. This is not called for.

Real changes in anybody's structure, including our own, generally take time to manifest in the functional and behavioral realms of experience. Consequently, we cannot expect to see anything change immediately in ourselves or anyone else. Moreover, we do not have to push anything through to its actual manifestation.

Sometimes we think it is our job to initiate something or to bring to someone else's attention the potential for change that exists in him or her. This is not so. Instead, it is up to each person to be enough in touch with him- or herself to become aware of the need to change, and to do something about it. For that matter, we should be too busy with our own inner work to get caught up in speculating about the changes we think somebody else ought to make.

We demonstrate our awareness of a need to change even when that need doesn't reach our conscious minds. Something in us will express this desire and we can then do what is appropriate to facilitate the process, whether in ourselves or in somebody else. As for what is "appropriate," this will depend on the person involved.

The psychological structures of this process are irrelevant. Whatever psychological states come to the surface only indicate that a person is alive and growing. We don't need to know anything else about it. For that matter, nothing else is really any of our business. Trying to decipher or discuss what something means can be just another way of intruding where we don't belong and of interpreting the situation for our own ends. Moreover, we always do so according to *our* level of understanding.

So psychological states have no necessary relationship to what is really happening. When we get caught up in them, we forget to pay attention to the deeper rhythm of an event. Better to keep it simple. We don't have to be aware of the psychological content of change but only of its rhythm. It might be useful to think about how a change could manifest, but even this is not necessary. Moreover, we have to be flexible in anticipating the particular process because we could be wrong about its outcome. Any mechanism can always take an unexpected turn.

It is important to understand that every person has his or her own internal program. Our job in any relationship is not to change anyone but only to support each other's unfolding. If we do it well, the whole situation will change, but according to its own inner logic. It may even come to the point where we recognize that our interests are diverging from those of the other person — but then, it was never our job to maintain a convergence of interests in the first place.

We have to learn to give to people as *they* want or need and not as we might want. There is no "ought" to this but only the reality of a person's own mechanism and whatever requirement he or she asks us to fulfill. If we cannot connect to others and convey that we genuinely respect and care for them in this way, then what are we as people? What are we demonstrating about our awareness of sacrifice?

As for what to do when others ask our advice, I generally try to avoid telling people what to do. I say this because we all ultimately do whatever we want anyway. Better to help the others in our lives do *that*, even if it leads to disaster. Then it is our job to be there and pick up the pieces — just as we hope others will do for us.

I may whisper what I think a person could try to do; I may even be full of suggestions at some point. Basically, however, I find it better to help someone do what he or she wants, even if I suspect it will end up in a train wreck. If somebody else wants to crash and burn, we have to let him or her do so.

After all, if a person *really* wants to go in that direction, there is nothing we can do. I have spent hours trying to convince people that what they were about to do was detrimental to their well-being. Rarely does it work. For that matter, people resent someone else's telling them what to do, which only puts us in a lose-lose situation.

What it comes down to, basically, is that nobody ever changes anybody else. Think about your response the last time somebody tried to change you. People change themselves. Anything that happens for a person is according to the logic and the mechanism within him or her. This is rarely related to the conscious mind, which has its own rate and direction.

More importantly, in many ways I don't even think that people really change, which is all the more reason why we are not here to change anyone. We cannot expect to kiss any toads and have them turn into Prince Charmings. We may just end up with bigger toads. Instead, we are all trying to find ways to be ourselves and looking for ways to mobilize our deepest potential. The secret is that this does not require us to be any different from who we truly are.

When People Leave

At the bottom of all service, sacrifice, and surrender is the recognition that Life Itself is free to do as it wills, and that every one of its manifestations is therefore an expression of that freedom. Put more basically, every person is inherently free. When we attune ourselves to the internal logic of another, and respect the particular way in which that logic is articulating itself, we are opening ourselves to that person's freedom, even when we do so at a cost to ourselves.

This is easy enough to say, of course, at least until the other person does something that we feel hurts us. Then we are challenged to listen at a deeper level for what is really trying to happen. For example, one of the hardest and most painful ways in which our lives call upon us to recognize the rhythm of change and to serve someone else's freedom is when he or she chooses to leave us. This confronts us with the question of what it really means to act from love.

Why do people come into our lives and why do they leave? I don't think there is any answer to this question or that we need to make any attempt to answer it. The fact is that people come. Some stay, some don't. It is really the energy speaking to the energy that is the issue here. Whatever walks out the door is not the essence of what we had.

In other words, the essence of the love that exists in our lives never walks out the door. It is always there. We just get some stupid ideas in our heads and, as a result, turn our backs on that living event that is the very source of our lives, the deeper love that manifests in many forms as we pass through this world.

The love in which we participate with other people is not intended to stick us together. We are here to share the work we have to do. That we are also able to share genuine respect and affection only demonstrates that we have our priorities straight. The minute we get stuck in it, however, then as one person stops being sweet the other one feels the need to react, and the whole thing becomes one great chain jerk. None of this is necessary.

As we grow, some things fall away. To refuse to let them do so violates the freedom of Life Itself and demonstrates cowardice on our part. Courage is necessary in spiritual growth. Letting go is never a comfortable process, no matter how often we do it. We have to be able to release anyone at a moment's notice. It is the only way to maintain our integrity and remain clear as to what we are about. It may seem as though we don't care, when in fact the opposite is the case. Sometimes, for example, my willingness to let people walk away has been taken as evidence that I am indifferent. Not at all.

If we are really growing, having anyone leave may hurt. However, it is also part of our liberation, and it clears the deck for new things. Nothing is ours to keep or change. Any idea we have that something was ours at any time is a fantasy. When anything leaves, it takes with it some of our illusions and delusions if we let it. If we fight the going, we are only holding on to these illusions. If we can allow it, the only thing we are really giving up is some stupidity. When people or things leave us, we always have two choices. We can get hysterical or we can get still. When we become entangled in the apparent multitude of outcomes to the situation, we only get confused, instead of recognizing that these are the only two real outcomes of any significance.

Like everything that is part of life, relationships have rhythms. They breathe, just as human beings do. The only problem is that most of us are so constricted that when a relationship tries to take a deep breath, we immediately react, perceiving it as a threat. So we take what is really a sign of life as a threat to our security. Then we go to war and end up killing the very living thing that we had. Of course, everybody likes to do that on some level because it is much easier to live with a corpse. Let's face it: you don't have to feed it, it doesn't give you grief, it makes minimal demands, and it stays just where you tell it to. Best of all, if you want to have a conversation, it doesn't talk back.

If we maintain the right balance in a relationship, there may be some fluctuation in the distance and closeness, but not much. Indeed, we enhance the possibility for constant attunement and intimacy even as we proceed with the work we are called to do in our daily lives. In practice we have to have everybody else's best interest in mind, not to the exclusion of our own but in terms of what is best for others and their growth. If we don't give them room to move, shift, and change, there will be little growth for anyone. To provide someone with this freedom, we must have established ourselves in a basic sense of inner well-being.

We cannot hold on too tightly to anything. It must have room to move around, and we have to learn to manage the discomfort this causes us. If we are going to demonstrate this process to anyone else, we had better be comfortable with it ourselves. Otherwise what are we communicating?

As we enter into any interaction, we want to be alert to our own tensions and able to eat them in the moment, in response to the needs of the situation. It is then necessary either to give up or just spin around and go 180 degrees in the other direction. This is not because it is a better direction but because it facilitates a flow. If we are stuck, we start by releasing what is stuck. We let go and surrender.

Maybe our minds want to pursue whatever is attempting to articulate its own freedom. Instead, we pause and become quiet. We don't hold on to the "I want something" issue but think instead, "What is the best for everybody here?" We choose to be a big person by releasing someone else into his or her own freedom even as we release yet another piece of our own limitation.

To Sustain a Subtle Distance

Is there any point at which we draw the line in extending the creative energy to facilitate a flow? It is true that as we move more deeply into our practice, we find that it becomes necessary to keep slightly apart from the people we love. This in no way means not loving them any longer; it doesn't mean not wanting to participate or share deeply in their lives. But if we are truly going to do our own inner work and facilitate this process in others, we cannot be fully extended into every situation. Otherwise we are likely to become off-center and reactionary.

First and foremost, we are concerned with and committed to practicing in order to develop ourselves. To the degree that we do this, we cannot help but experience something of a solitary life. Despite how this may sound, it is not a bad thing. The fact of the matter is that this is something that many people fail to discover about themselves: We all live solitary lives. Into this world we come alone, and alone we go out. In the middle there is love.

Our discovery of the unity of life and the infinite nature of our individualized self is not one we can make with other people. Rather we come to this vision, inspiration, and realization within ourselves. Then we carry it with us as we move in the world of manifold appearances.

It is not that we don't love others, but we cannot get seduced by that love or entangled in it. We have to keep some distance. Otherwise how can we be a true support to anyone else as their energy starts to shift and a transformation takes place? We will be chewed up in the transformation and the other person's respect for us will evaporate. Then there is no relationship, no matter how long the person endures in our company.

What I am suggesting is neither harsh nor cold. It is, instead, an appropriate distance that enables us to discern the rhythm of whatever we are interacting with, as well as the rhythm of any change that is taking place. It is this distance that allows us to reestablish our own balance and equilibrium. If we are really going to be of any assistance to anyone else, we have to be able to maintain this balance and equilibrium at all times. Paradoxically, it is the subtle distance we sustain that allows us to express a constant warmth. Without it, we burn out the situation and end up with a face full of ash. This then takes everyone no end of time to get over.

We can participate in the highest level of unity even as we move around in the world of diversity. Still, even as we move through this diversity we should not be confused about where we are. To sustain a subtle distance is another way of describing the process of keeping centered. When we are centered, we are not enmeshed in anything. Then from our own center we can relate to the center of everything else, at which point we can discover that this center, ultimately, is one.

Love

One of the most familiar Christian sayings, as Rudi used to point out, is that God is love. What we could add to this is that so are we. This kind of love has nothing to do with throwing ourselves at the feet of anything in worship. Rather it is our realization that our own, individualized nature is identical to the Self, which is love.

On one level this love is the energy that frees tensions. It is what enables the grace of the creative energy of Life Itself to flow without restraint. In our interactions with others, it is what requires that we find something to love within everyone we encounter. Love breaks down boundaries and barriers, including our judgments of others, because anyone who is alive is worthy of being loved. Simply to live is an act of creation.

When we cannot find a way to locate this love, we have to look to ourselves to find where we are wrong and to discover what we are doing to close ourselves off from the other person. Every tension we have with another person arises from some need within us to fight instead of opening ourselves and going further. It is nothing but a manifestation of our inability to transcend our egos.

We have to work to expand our energy. When there is any connection at all between us and somebody else, we have to do whatever we can to open and love them. What difference does it make what we have to do? If we cannot feel love, then we must sit down and work to open ourselves even further. This is important because if our energy does not manifest as love, it will express itself as some other kind of strong energy, namely, tension.

Nobody says we have to love everybody, but at least we have to see within ourselves what has to happen to help us open. Moreover, if we can assume full responsibility for the negativity we experience toward somebody else — if we can choose to eat the tension — then we can become aware of our real treatment of others. Even though their behavior toward us may not be entirely justified, we grow by recognizing what we fail to do for them. This is fully worth our effort.

Rudi used to say that nobody was enough for him to reject God. He said that when we let somebody come into our lives who distorts our sense of joy, they are taking us away from God. Nobody has the right to deprive us of that. But the responsibility to sustain that inner flow is ours alone.

There is a story about Nityananda and his ability to do this: One time in early spring when the mangoes were still ripening on the trees, a group of boys began throwing stones at the young fruit. Nityananda came out of the jungle, saw them doing so, and called to them to stop. Upon hearing him, the boys changed their target and began to throw their stones at him.

A strange thing happened next. Each stone that touched Nityananda fell to the ground as a sweet. The boys threw still more stones, and still more sweets fell to the ground. Without a word, Nityananda walked away and disappeared again into the jungle, while the boys ran to gather the sweets. This is how a saint behaves, giving sweets for stones.

We have to be able to encompass through love everything and everyone that comes into the field of our awareness. We have to open our hearts over and over again. When we can give of ourselves like this, we find that our need to do things in a restricted way will cease. It is this ability to open and extend ourselves to things as they are, and not as we would like them to be, that is unusual. It is to become a realist in the deepest sense — that is, of looking reality right in the eye because only there do we see God. There do we meet love.

This love is not a thing of the mind. Rather it arises from the spirit of our deepest inner Self and manifests through our hearts. Only in the later stages of our cultivation does it start to make sense to us in a real way; then our minds enter into it. Yet either way the power of the love we extend is phenomenal. The more we quiet ourselves and allow it to express itself and to work its magic around us, the more remarkable our lives become.

How does this relate back to what I said earlier about God and love being one and the same? I would shift this question a little and say, what is the relationship between universal love and surrender? Universal love is that fundamental conscious state from which all experience emerges and into which all experience subsides. It is love because it gives of itself continuously and asks nothing in return. It is pure giving, and its potential is infinite. So we call it love.

This universal love gives forth an infinity of form without ever being diminished in any way. The surrender of our individual boundaries, along with our limited ideas, hopes, and fears, is the vehicle by which we achieve an intimate, innate recognition of this same universal love within ourselves.

Rudi used to say that what we cannot surrender only becomes the resistance to our further growth. We could just as easily say that what we cannot give also obstructs our growth. To love something profoundly, to engage in it with intensity, and to be absorbed in it alone is sufficient for us to expand in a sense of total well-being. It is by this logic of love that we extend ourselves and in this love that we become established.

~~~~~~

The Shifts

*A man whose mind is merged in samadhi is not deluded
by the external magic show. He fears nothing, to him
there is no fear in the world. In his presence even the tiger
and the cobra forget their aggressiveness. All creatures
become calm. Even enemies forget their hostility and
become quiet. Why? There is no darkness then; the mind
is purified by pure light.*

— NITYANANDA

We have seen that the awareness of individual effort
characterizes the experience of the beginning student, while
the awareness of the energy characterizes the experience of
someone who has further refined his or her understanding.
The first person thinks of his or her interactions in the world as
exchanges of things and actions; the person with a more refined
understanding experiences those same events as exchanges of
energy. This leads to two important shifts in our awareness and
in the kinds of choices we make.

First of all, we become more aware of what facilitates
our awareness of the energy and what obstructs it. We also
become more interested in choosing the former and looking
for ways to transform the latter. This evolves into what we call
discrimination.

Second, we become increasingly aware of the power of Life Itself within us by allowing our old ways of seeing ourselves to fall away. Rather than clinging to our illusions about ourselves and others, we let them go. In the process, we face our deaths: We confront what is finite about us and what will die, even as we recognize what is infinite and beyond death entirely. Most of all, we understand our own relationship with the infinite and how this informs the life we are living now.

The person who faces these things is one who has internalized the understanding of sacrifice and who is so profoundly alive to the energy of Life Itself that he or she has gone beyond the fear of death. Such a person has released the limitations of his or her individual life, along with all concern for finite powers, surrendering them into the fire of the inner sacrifice and living immersed in the logic of love. Trika Yoga calls this person the *vira*, the "hero" or "warrior" — the person committed to living a heroic life.

These three things — discrimination, facing our death, and the vira — are all ways of talking about great shifts in our awareness. They deepen the understanding of shaktopaya even as they point beyond that awareness to something more subtle. As such, they are yet further refinements in our inner work.

DISCRIMINATION

Before their brains develop, babies see no difference in the world around them. It is only when their brains develop that the sense of difference develops. . . . A true yogi is like such a young baby. If you give the baby a diamond, he would throw it away; to him, a rock and a diamond are the same. Similarly, to a true jnani, a lump of earth and money are the same. He is not attached to either one. All is the Self; he sees the Self in all and all in the Self.

— NITYANANDA

What to Embrace, What to Avoid

Abhinavagupta, in one of his commentaries, starts out by discussing what we are to embrace in our lives and what we should avoid. The somewhat surprising thing is that he doesn't talk about any particular relationships or activities; he doesn't say we should avoid any forbidden things. Instead, he says quite simply that we must avoid all dualistic thinking and embrace the awareness that reality is one thing: consciousness, or the Self.

So he is saying that our spiritual work does not lead us to reject the world. After all, we cannot get away from it; nor do we want to. We do not deny or repress our awareness of any of the limited aspects of ourselves. Rather we learn to recognize this limited appearance to be an extension of something infinite. Therefore the issue is more subtle than a list of commandments or "Thou shalt not's." It is a matter of discrimination.

Everything we do and everything that happens to us acts as a source either of support or resistance to what we are trying to bring about in our lives at the deepest level. This is true of any specific life expression. The issue is always one of how we choose to take what we have done or what has happened and what we choose to make of it.

Here is the linchpin: The issue of discrimination arises in the context of decision-making. In any decision the real issue is one of understanding the big picture before us, perceiving the simple oneness underlying all appearance of diversity, and becoming centered in that awareness. When we have this in view, we see more clearly where we are going and what we have to do to get there.

Even here a process element is involved as we become established in that capacity for discrimination. Whatever we think we know today, we will forget tomorrow. For example, "being centered" will mean one thing to us now, and through simple shifts in our awareness, something quite different in a few years. However, when we understand this and still sustain our center steadily through all these shifts, then we intuitively know how to choose what will support our inner work. We know what is fitting.

I use the word "fitting" deliberately, because the issue of discrimination is not a matter of deciding that something is intrinsically right or wrong. It is not about being critical or judgmental. To be critical is an intellectual function, the more negative version of which is to be judgmental. When we judge something, we say, "*This* event looks like *that* one. Therefore they must be basically the same thing. I didn't like *that*, so I know I won't like *this*."

Such an approach may work in the most general sense, but more often it causes us to ignore details that may be important. Discrimination and judgment are two different things. If we look at a horse, for example, it can be black, white, or brown, or even a combination of all the above. To recognize the color of a horse in this way is called discrimination. If, however, we say that brown is good and black bad, that pink is good and white bad, or that all of the above are bad and we need a horse of different color entirely, then we are not only judging the thing but also making a mistake.

The real issue is discovering what uplifts our inner work. Some things are simply more effective than others. They work well, while others require a disproportionate amount of energy. So, we are talking about what works best and what doesn't work so well. We aspire to what works best because that is the most refined use and expression of our energy. One way simply gets things done more quickly, enabling us to go on to the next thing. That kind of creative flow allows for our participation in a much higher level of energy than does taking two years for the first thing, two years for the next, and so on.

There are, in other words, some laws here about the conservation and balance of energy: Balance and openness go together; judgment obstructs them both. To be judgmental is not balance nor is it real discrimination. The problem with judgment is that when we define something as either good or bad, we assume there is nothing more we can learn from it. If we think in terms of good or bad in the conventional sense, we end up right back in the dualistic soup.

Discrimination and Openness

The real source of discrimination is our experience of opening ourselves to the energy of Life Itself. Through our practice we experience over and over again what is really alive within us and, in the process, begin to recognize the vitality of that creative presence, not only *within* ourselves but flowing from us and back into us. We develop an awareness of what we are that is much more than this body and this broken radio between our ears.

Then discrimination requires no scientific definition, no long, sophisticated categories. In fact, with this kind of discrimination we will essentially be relieved of categories. This is not an intellectual activity or even an activity of the mind; rather it is a simple experience we have had over and over again so many times that we know it well and are able to let *it* guide our choices.

How does this express itself? On the most basic level, discrimination involves doing no harm. The next level enjoins us not to judge others. Third, we act not from a sense of rules or behavioral formulas, but with true insight into the nature of events, actions, and experience, in harmony with the creative power of the divine. We could also say in harmony with the creative energy, or with grace. Authentic discrimination involves seeing beyond all appearances and discerning the deeper reality inherent in every event. It requires that we be open.

In practice this is not so easy. Usually whatever we hope or expect to have happen obscures (or at least colors) our view of what is really going on. The force of our expectancy often leads us to overlook entirely the multiple possibilities inherent in any given moment.

And yet, infinite possibility is always present in every situation. Therefore we must be careful about what we close our minds to. Instead, we open our minds to every possibility, including totally outlandish ones. The *Maharthamanjari* gives examples of this by suggesting things that seem utterly impossible, such as the milking of birds.

The point is not to take such things as real but to open our minds beyond our own categories and judgments about reality. It teaches us to have some care in discerning the reality of what is manifesting before us instead of approaching it with closed minds that might overlook or deny the existence of something subtle and extraordinary. Openness of this kind then enhances our ability to recognize the depth in the actual reality presenting itself to us. This is the essence of discrimination.

What does this mean to us in a practical sense? For one thing, it means we come to recognize our internal dialogue as borscht, as only so many shredded beets. We also begin to understand, through the condition of openness that we cultivate in our practice, that there is only one real, authentic experience of Life, and that is surrender. Only in a state of surrender, in which our internal dialogue stops, can we participate completely in the infinity that we are.

Within every difficult period or moment that we face, we come into a junction point where we recognize that infinite possibilities exist. To know ourselves and be at peace allows us to appreciate the extraordinary rightness that can emerge out of such moments. What is wonderful within our lives can expand if we open ourselves and allow it to do so.

The wonderment described in some of the texts is that quality of openness that allows us to see what really *is* and that lets us rejoice in *that* without anticipating anything of our own construction. This wonderment emerges as we begin to understand that what is before us is infinitely more extraordinary than anything we could have possibly imagined. The elegance, grace, power, and breadth of Life's capacity for self-expression is, after all, truly extraordinary.

Then instead of trying to give birth to the baby *we* want to have, we give birth to the baby who wants to be born. Instead of trying to raise the child we imagine we need, we raise the child we actually have. Instead of imposing our will to create the person we think would make us happy, we support the person who has been created and who is actually emerging. We discover that person and, in the process, learn from, participate in, and appreciate even further the awesome power of Life Itself as it expresses itself in this particular form. Moreover, we do this in every context and situation.

If we are not open to the possibility of finding something wonderful and creative about everything we have ever been told is wrong, then we are in the wrong business. This is why, as we move through our lives every day, it is important to understand that in this practice there is no rejection of anything we are, any place we have been, or anything we are doing. These are not problems. We have to respect all the differences we find and learn from them, instead of rejecting or judging them. In that openness toward ourselves and others we find that all the appearances, including all the probabilities and improbabilities, can be reduced to a simple knowing that will sustain our contact with the creative potential inherent in any system.

Therefore this is the kind of discrimination that does not oppose anything. Nor does it mean we judge other people for whatever they have chosen to do with their lives. We can always find something to share. We understand that everything we see around us is simply Life. Moreover, we understand that what we think of as "good" is within us. When we cultivate and share that with everyone around us, we then find that there is good everywhere.

When we can do this, how do fear, doubt, self-denial, or self-rejection have any place in our understanding? We can begin to recognize when our minds hear something and grab hold of it. We can begin to discriminate between open and closed, between flowing and not flowing. These are subtle but powerful experiences. They are what will help us change our inner condition whenever we must.

To Keep Our Awareness Inside

I would like to come back for a moment to the notion that discrimination is not about rejecting the world. It is certainly true that much of our practice involves learning to keep our attention inside ourselves. However, some people have developed exotic ideas about what this means. They remove themselves from the world and develop disciplines such as not speaking for years, standing in strange positions for extended periods of time, or having no sexual contact.

Initially, such practices were probably aimed at helping people sustain their experience of inner intensification. At a certain point, though, this kind of asceticism becomes its own opposite and turns into the removal of all stimulus. It then becomes a kind of solitary confinement in which the person begins to fall apart from the inside.

When we speak of keeping our awareness inside, we must bear in mind that it is impossible to eliminate our external experience. It is neither necessary nor advisable to cut off all normal contact or interaction with the world. It is not even possible. Instead, we maintain ourselves in a state whereby our energy is always available to become established in the flow of our creative energy. Then we have not depleted ourselves in any way.

At the same time, if we are serious about this, we have to be careful to keep it simple. The potential to get lost in the vast quantity of stimuli around us is always there, as is the potential for confusion. It is analogous to the old scene of letting a child loose in a candy shop. This only creates the possibility for some kind of sickness, because a child may not know when to stop eating. For that matter, many adults don't, either. There is no point in filling ourselves with an overload of stimuli and then becoming constipated because we have poisoned our systems.

There are two extremes among people. One lives in an inner fantasy world; the other functions only in reaction to the world around him or her. Both are inappropriate approaches to experience, the attention of the one being artificially internalized, the other excessively externalized. Our interest in the creative energy transcends both modes because neither represents a case of keeping our awareness inside. Certainly, both demonstrate the absence of discrimination.

If we are ever going to deepen our spiritual search, we must ask ourselves often, "Is this thing or that relevant? Does it help me grow in the slightest?" Furthermore, what might be relevant information at some later date doesn't necessarily mean anything to us right now. We can tell ourselves it might be helpful in the future, but this is essentially ridiculous. If it will help at some point, then it will be around when we get there. These are determinations we can make effectively only as we learn more and more about what it means to keep our awareness inside.

Discrimination and Awareness of the Whole

True discrimination is awareness of the Self. When, through our commitment, we begin to arouse within ourselves a deeper contact with Life and cultivate that contact in both inner and outer realms, we start to see just what the subtle distinction between inner and outer really is. With that, the certainties upon which our lives have depended forever start to unravel. Consequently, discrimination also involves our recognition of where the boundaries between everything really lie — namely, in our own minds.

Which brings us back to Abhinavagupta's original point: What we embrace should uplift us. It should give us increasing access to, and broader participation in, the creative energy. Likewise, we avoid the thinking that causes us to identify with any of the various parts of this whole. We are enjoined, instead, always to understand that Life is an infinity. In understanding this we rise above every sense of ourselves as limited individuals.

Discrimination of this kind increasingly enables us to discern the shifts in frequency both within and around us. The stillness in the middle of these shifts allows for the unfoldment of a wondrousness that fills all space and transforms every form we encounter. When we have, and reside in, this awareness of the Self, we recognize that *everything* is to be surrendered. There is no further need to ask "Is this the Self, is that the Self?"

When we put our minds on one thing — that highest reality — we look at Life through the eyes of God. Then we understand what is compelling and essential to attend to and what is no more than crystallization. The fallout from the process of Life Itself has an intermediate existence that may be beautiful and even engaging, but it is still not anything on which to spend a lot of time.

True discrimination emerges only within a person who has a simple, broad frame of reference. Otherwise we become immersed in details, and our capacity for discrimination between one detail and another is overturned. This takes careful attention. It means we have to live our lives in a way that affords us the time, strength, energy, and clarity to turn our attention inside. It means we must have some awareness, so that we see whether or not things work out as we think they are supposed to. For example, if we don't have the effect on a particular situation that we expect, we must look both at what we did and at its outcome to see how to modify our approach.

Discrimination manifests itself in several ways of which we should be aware. In the first place, it expresses itself as acts of generosity. A person deeply aware of the energy of Life Itself as a whole is an actively generous person. Indeed, this is normal. To be in contact with the abundance that has created the whole universe, and to live from that awareness, brings an abundance into our lives that we cannot help but share in every way.

It also brings about the capacity for patient endurance. As we understand the nature of Life Itself more deeply, we recognize that, in fact, there *are* no real difficulties. Rather there are only different settings in which we unlock and release the energy crystallized in the material patterns that present themselves before us. These are just the many settings in which we allow that release to transform and renew our lives.

In our spiritual work we cultivate the qualities and the awareness that lead us, ultimately, to a capacity for the highest discrimination. It is this discrimination that changes the nature of our reason for growing. No longer do we do our inner work as a reaction against the brutality and stupidity of the world. Instead we recognize that something remarkable is hidden even within that stupidity and brutality.

Then we grow as an expression of our profound appreciation for all the magic hidden within all forms of Life, including all the stupidity and brutality. We see this magic within ourselves, each other, and all phases of the universe. At that stage, growing becomes a natural act of profound appreciation for the whole.

We breathe every moment and, in breathing, our bodies are renewed. Likewise, our capacity to be actively generous and to patiently endure revitalizes our total awareness of Life. Initially this is work and, as such, is in many ways a drudgery. In time, however, it becomes a joyous process. Then it is the patient acquisition, and endless sharing, of an extraordinary awareness.

This, too, is not so easy. It requires courage and the capacity to allow ourselves and our lives to change. So we practice this not only today but every day. If we come to recognize what is whole and living and what is dead within ourselves, and if every day we sweep away the dead, then before long we become fully alive, permeated with an understanding of infinite Life. Only our attachment to everything dead at the expense of the life within us causes us to get stuck in our own blindness.

It is our awareness of that dimension beyond all form and experience that allows us to be connected to the ever-newness of this pure Life Itself. Awareness makes us vehicles through which that newness finds its way into our ordinary lives. Our stability of mind and our devotion to that stability bring great richness into our lives. But it is discrimination that makes our perception of everything we encounter an act of worship.

Ultimately, discrimination is not what we do but the awareness and understanding with which we engage in our lives. Part of it is that we do whatever we do in a balanced way. The other part is that maybe we stop doing some of the things we now do. Every day we find our center, do what we have to do to sustain our awareness of the energy, and let the rest take care of itself. If we can live with that understanding and that degree of discrimination, then it is an easy thing.

I said earlier that surrender is the only authentic experience in life. We have also talked about surrender in many ways over the course of this longer discussion. What is the relationship between discrimination and surrender? Discrimination emerges from a condition of surrender. This is because surrender is a state of total openness in which we have released our attachment to our categories and judgments. It is the openness of pure potential. Surrender brings us into contact with that pure potential and allows us to become aware of how things unfold. It grows and grows the more we understand our experience of the creative process. Ultimately this is what discrimination is all about.

FACING OUR DEATH

When you know Truth, there is no fear of death. "I"
and "mine" are dissolved, "I" and "mine" are nothing
but fear of death. This is an obstruction on the path to
God. When you know Truth, death is just an external
condition, like sleep.

— NITYANANDA

Dying to Our Fear

One of my students, who happens to be a doctor, once
told me about a patient she had seen, a young man with a tattoo of a skull and crossbones on his arm. The tattoo read,
"Death is certain." Below that it read, "Life is not." Even
though the man may not have understood these words in a
particularly deep way, they were nonetheless true. Life is not
certain; death is.

Most people think about death at one point or another.
Certainly, the older we get the more we think about it. I
would even suspect that people think more about death than
about life. Often, it is only in retrospect that we think about
living. "Ho, ho, ho, remember the time . . . ? Boy, *that* was
really living!" Either that, or we think about life in terms of
our various difficulties and reasons for worrying.

When we look at any of these issues more carefully, we
can usually find ways to go beyond our particular concerns for
what will happen to us in any given situation. Nevertheless,
we still confront the big one: Ultimately, the mantra of stupidity ends up being a question about what will happen to us
when we die. Extensions of this idea appear in questions like
"What will happen to me after my body dies? Will I go on?
Does consciousness endure?"

Ironically, death doesn't bother us all that much in other
contexts. We watch nature programs on television and see the
cheetah killing the antelope or the lion jumping something
else, while a commentator describes the whole thing for us
blow by bloody blow. We don't object to these creatures killing

each other for food, nor do we find their deaths deeply disturbing. We find it easy, however, to become highly emotional about death when it involves people. Sometimes I wonder why.

That I focus on death like this may lead you to think I am being morbid. I am not. If I talk about dying it is because it is important to face the fact that everybody does it; none of us avoids it. The fear that comes upon us when we think about this is based on our lack of understanding about who we are and what death really is.

For one thing, we misunderstand the power that Life *is* within us: the power that motivates this mass of solids and that causes us to struggle in the world, to suffer, be afraid, feel pain, chase solutions, and hold on to things. All this is caused by our misunderstanding of what we are, making our fear of death and our attachment to survival in the physical sense intensely powerful.

I would suggest that it is because of our limited understanding and attachment to the forms of experience we know (in other words, because of a lack of discrimination) that we have no access to the substance of experience. We do not recognize the vast, creative vitality implicit in all experience or the universal power from which experience arises. This makes it difficult for us to go beyond our concern for the momentary forms.

Whatever we fear rules us. The more we give that fear credence or even attention, the more it governs our lives. Just as the more we create excuses for not being happy the more these excuses become our masters, so our fear becomes our ruler and our master. Indeed, for most people, fear is their god and they pray to it every day not to bite them.

One of the reasons for this fear is that when we talk about "life," we usually mean "my life." More specifically, when we say "life," what we really have in mind is this body, or "my life, in this body." Many people have the basic suspicion that we are conscious only because we have bodies. Yet your life and your body are not the same thing. For example, you may be a part of my life, but you are not my body. My life is much more than my own body or any other part of my experience.

Suppose you see a powerful, concentrated energy event moving along the ground — say, a tornado. If it were not for its picking up a lot of dust and other material debris that organize themselves into that funnel, we would not be able to see it because it is really only a great current of energy.

Likewise, the energy event that we are gathers around itself various kinds of organic matter, something like that dust and debris. Our body is a chemical envelope, and each and every one of its chemicals has energy as a basis. When the particular form of this energy event dissipates, the dust and debris also dissipate and fall away. That doesn't mean the energy is gone; indeed, we know from the work of many scientists over the last fifty years that energy is never destroyed.

When a person dies we ask, "What happened?" Then we say things like "Well, he had a heart attack and since no air was getting to the cells, he died." We say, "A fuse blew. There was a disruption in the power to the main circuits and, consequently, the message telling the heart to beat didn't make it. Then the lights went out." We say many different things about the cause of death, but we still cannot really say what happened.

According to the Trika Yoga perspective, on the other hand, there is no such thing as death. Our bodies may die as unified organisms, but even these, when they decompose, remain organic matter that can nourish other organic matter. What is alive within us is always alive; what dies are our illusions. This is what becomes clear to us the more intimately we come to know the nature of the energy that is the source of our lives.

When Rudi passed away, his family asked me to go to the funeral home after his body had been brought there, to see that everything had been done properly. I was told I had to look at the body, so I did. What could I say? It looked like Rudi, but nothing about that body had anything to do with what Rudi is, was, or ever had been. My point is that whatever dies was never truly alive in the first place, so how can we call it "life?" And if that is so, then what, in the deepest sense, is there to fear about death?

Our practice enables us to recognize this and be quiet with it. There is no need for us to negate the pain of our experiences. It is simply part of living. What we would like to do, instead, is establish ourselves in the finest vibration within ourselves and maintain that stability, irrespective of the circumstances. Then, whether we feel pain or pleasure, we are not drawing back from or reaching out toward either one, but are centered and encompassing the pulse of our own awareness and unfoldment.

Rudi passed away a long time ago. I loved him completely. He was the source of my life, and he left. Still, through that whole experience of his death, I never felt one moment of sadness. To some degree this surprised me. But real love does not die. As we grow and change, our experience and understanding of love, and therefore of death, are transformed. There is no longer a kind of dependency, no longer any attachment involved in it, and nothing to fear in its change of state.

Somebody once asked me, "If you were in a political situation in which somebody came to you and said, 'Do this terrible thing or we will kill you,' what would you do?" I said, "I would have to say, 'Kill me. It would be better than living under someone like you.'" This is how I feel about the fear of dying. If fear came and threatened to kill me, I would have to say, "Kill me, then. It is better than living under you." Better to die than to live with fear. If we take the fear, greed, lust, tension, and everything else from which human beings function in this world — if we take all that and hold it up in front of the mirror of death — we see that every bit of it is worth less than dung.

It is better just to face our deaths and accept the fear. Not reacting, clenching, or losing our concentration, we hold our center and our happiness, even when it does actually mean dying. When we can face our fear and project it out to its logical extreme, it becomes ridiculous. Since it is the fear of death that really kills us, why not die within ourselves to that fear now and get it over with? Then we can be happy no matter what is happening in our lives. The point is this: If the Self is the source of everything, and every aspect of our experience is nothing but a mode of the Self, then even death and decay cease to be frightening. How can they be, when we ourselves are the Self of death?

In the Mirror of Death

People practice martial arts for years to develop the capacity to remain completely centered and calm in the face of truly life-threatening situations. Our practice prepares us in similar ways. Instead of becoming hysterical in the face of death, we become quiet and ready to dance, if need be. This is why it is a good thing to practice steadily, cultivating and refining our awareness of our center and our sense of the flow within and around us. In this way we dissolve our resistance and absorb from our environment the subtle information of which we may not be overtly aware.

Only when we begin in earnest and with great dedication to pursue our understanding of what it means to have a direct connection to Life Itself; only when we make the effort to take down the walls — to break, penetrate, and dissolve our tensions, to rise above our patterns and extend our awareness throughout the whole field of this creative experience — only then do we begin to live authentically. Then we experience pain, anguish, and suffering directly, and die for a real reason.

I will tell you something else. The greatest amount of energy we will ever be called to absorb in our whole lives will be at the moment of our death. This is why it was believed in ancient Chinese biographies that the quality of a person's life is disclosed by the manner in which he or she faces death. If we have not prepared ourselves to face it with equanimity, the experience will sling us around severely.

On the other hand, when we make a commitment to grow we will, as a part of the process, accept and come to terms with death early on. That is, we will begin to understand what it really means to say that what is alive in us now is always alive, while what dies was never alive in the first place.

When we understand that we are not as tightly composed and readily identifiable as we once thought we were, we are more able to relax about the notion of dying and to pay more careful attention to the process by which we *are*. If death is not such an issue, then what *are* we? If our body is not an issue, then what is? These are questions in which any thoughtful human being would take an interest if we were not so afraid of what has to happen first.

By developing the capacity to remain in contact with the various resonances of which we are composed and which are really a series of overlapping fields of vibration, we come to look upon our individuality and our mortality much differently. We are no longer threatened by the ongoing changes in our composition as we become aware of them. Only when we are able to see beyond the chemicals, however, can we understand that our reaction is not reasonable. Seeing beyond our physical bodies to the energy that motivates and sustains them puts an end to our preconceived notions of dying.

Once we see the superficiality of our physical existence and all the things that go along with that, such as our pursuit of comfort and satisfaction, our vision changes. Basically, the drama disappears. After all, if we know ourselves, then how can death appall us? We stop asking, "What's going to happen to me? How am I going to avoid dying?"

We no longer see ourselves as bodies, or as events in need of anything. Once we are no longer clinging to our bodies, we are able to be good friends with death. We might even hang out with death from time to time; you never know. Not only that: We are able to look beyond our bodies, minds, and emotions, and beyond our profoundly limited interests, to see ourselves as connected to a vast and awesome creative power. We see that we are a part of it, just as it is a part of us.

Further, it reveals all our bodily and worldly concerns to be pure ignorance. Held up to the mirror of death, our material life is a sea gull dropping on the surface of the ocean. If we understand that Life Itself is infinite — that what is alive is alive and, by definition, does not die — then fear, doubt, insecurity, and suffering no longer have any hold on us.

Death and Rebirth

In my view, we have all died more than once already in this life. This is true on a number of levels. First of all, every seven years the cell population of our bodies turns over completely. This means that from period to period in our lives we are chemically not the same person. If we look back, there are also certain experiences we can refer to as so profoundly transforming that we might say the person we were actually died.

If this is true in our ordinary lives, it is all the more true of our spiritual work. This is represented in the ceremony for becoming a swami, which entails three days of death rituals. The last of these is the death ritual one performs for oneself. At that point, the person one was ceases to exist and is ritually burned. Then he or she goes forward with a new name. This name is not that of a person, but of a quality of universal consciousness. So even though the appearance of some individuality is there, it becomes incidental. This death erases its power and there is only the apprehension of the underlying power of Life Itself.

From either perspective, death has happened to all of us more than once, and it is no big deal. We emerge from our encounter with it bearing more or fewer scars, depending upon the nature of our awareness as we move through it. When we experience it as painful, it is usually because we are so busy holding on to what is being taken out of the right hand that we don't see what is being given to us in the left.

There is also a growing body of research on near-death experiences showing that some people have actually experienced moving through that veil and then back again. However we view these experiences, they do occur. Furthermore, in our spiritual work we will have similar experiences. In meditation people often report such things as moving back and forth between this body and world and other worlds, as well as seeing other people at great distances and going even beyond that. Life and death as we usually think of them are simply not the limits we imagine.

The most powerful experiences of life available to most people are those related to birth and death. The similarity between the two is remarkable. I have never gone through birth from the perspective of a mother, but having been an observer at both birth and death, it seems to me that they are not all that different. Both are changes of state. For that matter, the experience of life is also an experience of the process of dying, because death is implicit in every moment of our lives.

Whatever a mother thinks about during pregnancy pre-occupies her child in some way for at least the first thirty years of his or her life. Similarly, whatever is on our minds when we die is on our minds for a long time after that and can easily become the vibration around which a whole new life develops. Moreover, our experience of death is basically an extension of how we have lived. People who are already at peace with themselves don't worry all that much about dying.

This suggests that we always have to be ready to let go of everything and everybody. Ultimately, we will have to do that anyway, but we start with our own bodies. Better to get used to that idea sooner rather than later, because if we wait until the last minute, it becomes almost impossible.

This process is not easy, because as we let go of one attachment after another, each little death can be accompanied by the falling away of people and situations who have been a part of our nourishment and support. As we change, these people may no longer choose to be a part of our lives. This can make us want to cling to what is familiar, even if it means settling for a kind of death in life.

Yet from a certain perspective, we are already dead. The issue is only one of when, not if. In this sense, our fate is already sealed. Life here is only a truck stop, and in the biggest possible picture, the food is not much better than what we find at any other truck stop. Furthermore, even if our entire lives were somehow wiped out, they would still be restored. Maybe not immediately, but everything in our lives could go away and it would all basically come back in a renewed form. Cut the grass and it grows back. Chop down trees and they send up new shoots. As for weeds, there is no getting rid of them.

There is a further way of looking at it: How often do we return to the places we have left? From the point of view of most of the people we have left behind, we are dead. They don't see us or know anything about us, so as far as their lives are concerned, we have died. I suppose we could say that this makes wherever we are now heaven. Leaving life as we know it is the same thing. There is nothing to fear, and so nothing to resist. It is simply a wonderful circumstance to be embraced at the proper moment.

In Rudi's writing, and certainly in his talks, we hear the same point: It is necessary in a very real way to die and be reborn. Moreover, this must happen not just once or twice but often. Every human being is an expression of the divine, just as all the things we do and all the things that happen to us are extensions of that same divine. This includes our dying.

This revelation takes place from within ourselves. It is not that someone whispers it in our ear, but that our own hearts disclose it to us. If we are not quiet we will never hear it. This requires that we open ourselves to our pain, distress, disappointment, and struggle. It means that maybe we die to our fear in order to conquer our senses, master ourselves, and be reborn into authentic life, growing beyond the constraints of the person we were.

Unless we can release over and over again everything we have received in life, we will never be free. Rudi once said that only when we see the deepest and most meaningful of our possessions taken away can we understand the whole process as a manifestation of the mind. It is only our grieving, he said, that brings about the loss.

We are all going to die; we just don't know when. In a way it really doesn't matter when or how. My only feeling about it is that in dying, it helps if we can relax, and even more if we can concentrate. It is better to die consciously, releasing into the experience, in order to pay attention to the flow.

Never Closer to Eternity

Trika Yoga suggests that the mind is a reflection of, or in some way similar to, the highest consciousness. It is said that only after the body ceases to exist does a person become that highest consciousness with no sense of differentiation in the slightest. This tells us something about the attitude of the Trika philosophers toward death: that when our bodies cease to exist, we finally recognize and become fully established in that utter and complete understanding of our intimate condition as the highest reality.

They were not suggesting that this is automatic. The lives of many people represent such dense contractions of tension and crystallization that the possibility for release upon death is minimal — not non-existent, but minimal. Again, our experience of moving through death is highly colored by the resonance that we have established in our minds over the course of our lives.

Still, the point is that whether we live or die, the consciousness that is the foundational power of Life Itself is not two, but one. When we recognize that oneness and start to experience it as a palpable presence asserting itself from within us, when our minds become still and we watch them long enough to understand them somewhat, then the notion of death becomes irrelevant.

When we have this attitude, the work we do and the actions in which we engage are not done out of a sense of obligation or guilt toward our parents, our ancestors, or society. We continue to act in the world, but do so from a sense of love, appreciation, joy, and respect for Life Itself.

The brother of one of my students once said to me, "I've been thinking that we are never closer to death than we are right this minute. But doesn't that mean that we are also never closer to eternity than we are at this moment?" Life Itself is an infinity. So there is no one moment when we are closer to, or farther away from, any part of it than we are at any other moment in our lives. We are unified with the whole at all times. Finding that unity makes for a great change in our vision of things because if there is only one thing, only one power, then we do not have to worry about what happens to us when these bodies fall apart. Life simply persists.

At that point we are able to look upon the whole world as nothing but that creative process happening in us. In this shift we find and experience the infinite resource within ourselves even as we begin to understand our nearly limitless creative capacity. We find complete peace and the experience of total well-being. In this shift we become nonattached. The importance of this is the reason I talk about death a fair amount.

We are able to relax and, with virtue, generosity, patience, and sustained effort, cultivate within ourselves the capacity for contemplative attention and discriminating awareness. These then allow us to recognize all superficial boundaries, first extending them, then finally dissolving them insofar as they limit our awareness and the structure of our own being. This frees us to participate completely in the experience of authentic living.

Then our actual experience of this authenticity and our understanding of the vastness of Life Itself remove us from the realm of suffering. We come to a real experience and tangible understanding of what the end of this process is about. We understand where it comes from and where it ends, which is in infinity, or eternity. We also recognize that at this very moment we *are* as close to eternity as we can be. There is no moment when we will ever be closer.

The Heroic Life

To whom pain and pleasure are equal, who is
self-contained,
To whom a clod, a stone and gold are the same,
To whom the loved and the unloved are equivalent,
who is steadfast,
To whom blame and praise of himself are alike,
To whom honor and dishonor are equal;
Dispassionate toward the side of friend or foe,
Renouncing all undertakings,
He is said to transcend the gunas.

— THE BHAGAVAD GITA

The Mastery of the Vira

The discussion of discrimination and of facing our death brings us to the idea of the vira. This term means "hero," or "warrior." The image of a warrior may be one that we ourselves have a hard time relating to, particularly if we associate it with our perceptions of military life. I am talking, however, about something very different. The term "vira," to the Trika masters, was a way of describing a state of awareness.

To us this may seem like a strange way of talking about a warrior, but in the Trika tradition it refers to the person who has fully internalized the awareness of shaktopaya. This is someone who is profoundly alive to the awareness of the energy in all phases of his or her experience. The vira is a person who has come to embody the spirit of the sacrifice and whose whole life is an articulation of the logic of love.

The image of the warrior finds various expressions in different parts of Asia. Some of the most poignant stories that come out of East Asian culture, for example, are those of the *ronin* of Japan; the samurai who has lost his lord, or whose lord has fallen. These people were proud, skilled human beings who were thrown onto the street to live with only their dignity. Indeed, the ones with dignity suffered the most because there was no status in being a soldier without a lord. (The ranks of the unemployed are looked down upon everywhere.) A ronin with no real place to use his skill either turned to banditry or starved. The worst became criminals.

I sometimes imagine that a similar class of people must have existed in India. It occurs to me that some of the early ascetics and wanderers may have emerged from the ranks of such warriors, and from years of experience on the battlefield. I imagine, for example, the training that warriors in India had to undergo to prepare themselves to enter into battle. In fact, there are sects of the *dasanami* order that are warrior monks. They existed in greater numbers in the past, but are extant even today.

We find graphic portrayals of the warrior in India in the epic *The Mahabharata*. Imagine, afterwards, being forced to roam about India and fend for yourself. Would it be surprising that some of the spiritual practices of the wandering ascetics arose in part from such experiences? It might give us some sense of the logic that accompanied the emergence of these things.

A warrior of this class was dedicated, in one sense, to his own survival. However, he also dedicated his life to a greater purpose. In the service of this greater purpose he faced the possibility of losing his own life. There was thus a strong incentive to develop his technique and become skillful in the martial arts. Indeed, he concentrated on developing these skills as the means to his salvation in the moments when he was called upon to serve that higher purpose.

There was a certain dedication — and, in the best of warriors, a strong devotion — implicit in what made a warrior what he was. Yet, no matter how skillful one became, going out onto the battlefield was still a chaotic event, with people hacking away at each other with pikes and swords. Moreover, whether the setting is ancient or modern, a warrior faces chaos and uncertainty. This is not merely the uncertainty of a backgammon game where the issue is one of which dice we will roll. Instead, it is a matter of blood and rolling heads.

The strain implicit in the existence of the warrior required a strong mastery of the mind and senses. First and foremost, the warrior had to take responsibility for his own life, not blaming anybody else and not being all that concerned with the ebb and flow of life's forces. The true vira had gone beyond being absorbed by the question "What's going to happen to me?" Thus, in Kashmir Shaivism, vira does not mean "warrior" or "hero" in the way we may assume; rather it means one who has cut away all doubts and mastered him- or herself.

From the point of view of the writers of Shaivism, there are essentially three levels of people who participate in the endeavor of spiritual work. The first are devotees, or beginning students. The second are the viras. The third are known as *siddhas*, or perfected ones. These distinctions correspond to the three phases of our practice.

Devotees participate in, and recognize, only duality. They see things in terms of teacher and student, subject and object. Where they are is where they want to go: Beginning from the pursuit of desire, ambition, and the need for attainment, they see their spiritual work from this perspective. That is, they practice with the hope of getting something in return. This is normal. At the same time, the inner work of the beginning student lies in going beyond these concerns.

The vira is a person who understands sacrifice deeply, a person who has transcended his or her desires, ambitions, and objectives and who participates in a universe of creative energy in which he or she recognizes life and individual experience as an extension of the flow of infinite Life. Such a person is called a hero because, in every case, he or she has surrendered personal boundaries, risked personal safety, and risen above personal imperatives in order to benefit the whole. Such a person, in so doing, experiences him- or herself to be more than the boundaries of what is individual.

This is what we admire about a hero. This is someone who has faced danger and risked him- or herself for the safety and welfare of others, who has the capacity to put the needs of others before his or her own. The term vira refers, therefore, to a person who in many ways has mastered him- or herself to that heroic extent. This is a person who functions from an awareness of a higher interest.

In the Spirit of the Sacrifice

What bearing does this have on our own work? At some stage we recognize that the pressure we absorb is nothing other than energy. Seeing this enables us to look beyond the limits of our egos to face our own death. When we are able to do this, a different logic starts to function in our lives.

I referred earlier to this as the logic of love, but we can also talk about it in terms of attaining the awareness of the vira, in which we experience ourselves as participants in a vast, dynamic event. We find we have the capacity to participate in circumstances at great distances from us simply by being aware of, and understanding, the way the total network functions. At that point our definition of "self-interest" expands enormously.

A person who can do this is one who is also capable of functioning under great stress while keeping clearly in focus what will benefit the whole. This is a person whose interest lies in knowing the infinite and knowing God. One who qualifies as a vira, an advanced student, is one who wants to know that transcendent state. It is not someone concerned with making money, getting ahead, or even with solving problems.

This is a person who lives in the spirit of the sacrifice. It is someone trained to live a life of functioning under pressure, under conditions that would paralyze an ordinary person. Anybody can enter into the sacrifice, but only those who can endure it remain. These are the viras, who function for the benefit of the world.

A vira is a person who transcends him- or herself. The arena in which this happens does not much matter. The vira is capable of recognizing his or her own fear, weakness, selfishness, and self-absorption and is able to set all that aside in order to serve the legitimate needs of other people, often at his or her own expense. Our self-respect and the respect of others grows based on our capacity to embody these things: to transcend ourselves at any given moment, discover what the situation requires, and give it.

This describes a person who has surrendered control of his or her life and, in the process, has also surrendered the limitations of that life. In many ways this is a person who takes responsibility for his or her own actions and who accepts the consequences of those actions. Most of us aren't even aware of the consequences, let alone of having accepted them, but this is one of the meanings of transcending our actions. This is the sacrifice of the small self.

We might say, therefore, that the vira is detached. This is a little tricky because the term "detachment" can suggest that a person is uncaring. This is not the case. I would say, instead, that one who is detached is centered, able not to give a great deal of importance to the short term and not to worry too much about what others think. The ability to do this has everything to do with the character of one's awareness, which is what one chooses it to be.

From an objective point of view, it doesn't matter how other people judge us. What matters is the intensity of our own participation in the moment, in awareness of the rhythm of the Self. A warrior with this awareness can find him- or herself in the middle of battle and remain unconcerned about the surrounding circumstances. Not involved in whether he or she is going to live or die, the warrior is simply there, one-pointedly dealing with what awaits doing. Indeed, living and dying are not the primary questions on the mind of such a person.

For that matter, the question "What's going to happen to me?" is also not at the forefront of such a person's awareness. "What's going to happen to me?" is already a foregone conclusion: We are going to die no matter what. As I said earlier, the issue is not if but only when. Knowing that, we try to be one-pointed on the moment and focus on it. We develop the capacity to do so by training ourselves to focus on every level of our breath. The bottom line over and over again is to keep it simple and do our own work.

Even as we take responsibility for our lives, we have to be able to share them with others in a sharing neither based on need nor predicated on the business of relationships or of wanting anything from anybody else. We see beautiful, admirable, and inspiring things in the people around us, and we celebrate them. We can even say that we worship those wonderful things. Likewise, we celebrate that which is terrifying. We celebrate it all.

The Only Heroic Quest

Two things accompany the warrior: torture and death — and they don't necessarily go together. In one sense, it is not a happy situation, given that the choices are pretty grim. Yet there is a certain exhilaration involved in facing extraordinary challenges and in participating, even succeeding, in these events with intense clarity. This makes it irrelevant whether we win or lose. The outcome becomes unimportant.

A battle is an event that brings some soldiers either to the discovery of their own cowardice or to their deaths. This same event can also allow the inner greatness of others to be recognized. What brings an ordinary person lower can be the occasion for a fine person to become finer. Any challenge, and all difficulty, involves sacrifice. It is the testing ground of the vira.

So we have to have the capacity to concentrate one-pointedly on what we are doing, step by step, without getting lost. In the heat of battle we have a job to do, and we have to concentrate in order to accomplish it. We cannot bother with what is going on over on the other side of the field; we have our own work. We have to do it with vigor and enthusiasm, yet with resignation.

The story of *The Bhagavad Gita*, in which the warrior Arjuna questions the purpose of going into battle with his kinsmen, is a meaningful text in this regard. Arjuna's charioteer, who is in reality the god Krishna, answers him by discussing the means by which a person can develop within him- or herself the strength of spirit, as well as the inner centeredness and quiet, necessary to march into battle without being afraid. From that inner strength we discover that there is no need to worry about winning or losing, about surviving or dying. We just go in and do what we must. That is a powerful state.

We become aware that we are part of a living medium — that everything we touch and relate to is essentially nothing but the same essence that we ourselves are. As we become aware of these more subtle levels of vibration, we find that they have a kind of infinity to them because they are not centered anywhere. Rather they exist as the very foundation of all spatial, temporal structures. We slowly start to recognize the infinite nature of our individual awareness.

It is not only because we reach for this awareness but also because of how we experience it that we rise to the status of vira. We attain the inner strength and awareness that enable us to transcend our self-interest and, in so doing, to have our self-interest maximized. How does that happen? As we transcend our petty self-interest, we become a bigger vessel, through which our self-interest is expanded, unfolded, and fulfilled. We become bigger people by giving of ourselves. Because of our surrender, which emerges out of the recognition that even the greatest of warriors dies, we are comfortable and even full of wonder in our constant contact with that infinity.

We are out to slay the dragon of the mind. This is, ultimately, the only heroic quest that exists for any human being. However we rise to the level of the heroic within us it is specifically because, and only because, we engage that limited aspect of ourselves and transcend our fear within the context of some intense and potentially life-threatening circumstance.

Whenever a person is recognized to have become a hero, it is because he or she has addressed some limited aspect of him- or herself and defeated it. Whether it be in actual battle or in the quest to transcend the limitations inherent in the mind, the challenge remains fundamentally the same. The dangers of the latter, if anything, are more subtle and potentially more insidious because we have little built-in bias against the mind. Its dangers are not so obvious on the front side.

Our search for the hero within ourselves requires us to confront all our fears, scruples, and feelings toward the things that repulse us. It calls us to rise above all that. Instead, we must have the capacity to find ourselves in unusual and difficult circumstances and maintain our equilibrium.

The endeavor as a whole releases us from characterizations of ourselves as female or male, old or young, smart or stupid, wealthy or poor. All such discussions no longer apply to a person who has achieved the status of the heroic within him- or herself. There is only, each day, the process of confronting every boundary that asserts itself within our lives.

By our commitment and by the power of the breath within us, we transcend these boundaries and extend our awareness to the limit of our own essence. There, we discover, there is no limit. In this is all our freedom.

Shambhavopaya

By union with the collective whole of all the energies, through intensive and fixed awareness, there is the disappearance of the universe as something separate from consciousness.

— SHIVA SUTRAS

Introduction

Individual and Universal Consciousness

Having been brought up a Christian, when I left Christianity behind I had many doubts about whether or not there was such a thing as God. Even well after I met Rudi I remained uncomfortable with the use of the term. I think this was partially because of my feelings about my Catholic background and partially because it had not been my experience to know directly that there was such a thing.

In the intervening years, however, it has become clear to me that, in fact, God *is*. This has nothing to do with any concept of God drummed into me as I was growing up; it has nothing to do with someone to whom we pray or petition for one thing or another. Rather it has everything to do with experience that comes out of spiritual practice.

Both the Bible and the different Tantras say that the human being is a microcosm of the universe. The Bible says we are made in the image of God; the Tantras say we are a microcosm of the macrocosm. In Western culture this has often led people to think of God in human terms, something like a great person who has a mind with its own program and ego. In India the tendency has also been to personify the divine and project that divinity onto many forms.

Both approaches have some merit for a certain phase in our spiritual work. At the same time, it is easy in both cases to profane the discussion — to see the infinite in our own image and more or less justify our life programs from that perspective. This leads people into doing every kind of horrible, knee-jerk, reactionary activity imaginable, all in the name of God. Moreover, when we think about Life as a whole, we tend to assume that whole to be like *our* lives as we know them. This is another way of reducing the divine to a level on which God has two eyes and ears and acts like a dummy, instead of elevating ourselves to understand just what God is.

This tendency is not readily overcome, because the nature of reality is so much more sophisticated. It is easier to let our understanding of God be shaped by the way we live than to allow that understanding to be transformed as we surrender our tensions and desires, recognize the infinite creative energy at work in all things, and from that experience, have some awareness of our own essential foundation.

One of the important ideas in Kashmir Shaivism is that there is nothing exterior to God, or consciousness. The first aphorism in the *Shiva Sutras* says, "The Absolute has, as its nature, consciousness." From the point of view of shambhavopaya, ultimate reality is pure, vital consciousness. We could also say pure, conscious energy.

There are hundreds of names for this. Sometimes we refer to it as the Self, sometimes as creative energy. I call it dynamic stillness. They are all the same thing, and they are all ways of talking about God. The different words imply different emphases. They suggest shifts of focus just as we, in moving through our lives, continuously shift focus. Still, consciousness is both one and universal. It is neither separate nor distinct from anything.

Every individual spirit has as its essence this nature of universal consciousness. Thus our individualized consciousness is intimately and directly related to infinite consciousness. The ancient philosophers of India put it succinctly in saying that God is consciousness, or that consciousness is God. It must be, therefore, that God is somehow related to our own consciousness.

Without the experience of an interaction between our consciousness and the highest awareness, how could we intuit the latter? Indeed, even to suggest that there is such a thing as God requires some basis in experience. Otherwise from where would the idea come? Nor is this a conjectured unity. Rather through the experience of our inner work it is discerned to be living and dynamic, and thereby in keeping with the nature of universal reality.

So the energy of our inner Self is two things. It is at once the most intimate and personal part of what we are; at the same time, it is also universal and transcendent. Moreover, there is a continuous, reciprocal relationship between the individual and the divine, between the intimate and the transcendent. Yet there is no point where individual and universal consciousness separate.

In short, we experience nothing outside of consciousness. Although our individuality is not separate from it, consciousness is still greater than all the contracted aspects we take on. This suggests that only from the perspective of Life Itself can our individual existence truly be examined and understood.

Ultimately, to say that our individual consciousness and universal consciousness are one defines our inner work as the examination of that greater consciousness. As we meditate and do this work, we develop a capacity independent of our senses and free of our bodies that enables us to appreciate the consciousness at the core of our existence. From the experience of the infinity of Life — the infinite, formless presence of the divine — we have the opportunity to turn around and reflect again upon what we take to be "I."

The first point is to have a palpable contact with the energy of Life Itself. We find that the strongest experience of that energy resides in the intimate expression of "I." This is the power of consciousness demonstrating itself. Think about it: When we say "I," we are not really talking about our bodies, thoughts, or feelings. We may say, "I think," "I feel," but the experience of the "I" is always first, after which that "I" does something. Moses quoted God as saying, "I am that I am."

When you or I refer to "I," are we talking about something different? There may be the appearance of a uniqueness, and if we are talking about our bodies, there is the appearance of distinction. Likewise, each mind is somewhat different. Yet the "I" we all speak of doesn't refer to these things but to consciousness, which is not the individual mind. Although our minds are contained in it, *it* cannot be contained by the mind. Nor is it our emotions, though it contains these, too. It is greater than our individuality, and yet it contains our individuality.

The true "I" is an awareness from and to which we speak. It is an effulgence, a pulse, an energy. When our awareness is centered and stabilized in that energy, then the rest of the field takes on its proper perspective.

What then do we observe? The one thing we all have in common is consciousness, the most mysterious and subtle phenomenon in the universe. What does consciousnesss observe but itself? Wherever you focus, it is really only one thing. Then, appearances notwithstanding, subject and object remain undifferentiated. There is no distinct object but only subject. Indeed, every act of cognition is possible only because of a preexisting relationship to the subject. That relationship is one of consciousness, in which consciousness is simultaneously the knower, the known, and the process of knowing.

Forgetting the Individual

When Rudi said that true spiritual growth involves the destruction of the self, he was referring to the structure of our individuality. In this regard, it is not that we set out to destroy anything. Rather we make the effort to bring the extraordinary power and creativity within us to the forefront of our awareness. In recognizing the infinity of our spiritual richness, the poverty of our individuality also becomes apparent. We don't cease to exist; we do cease to be the same person we were. A transformation occurs in which we recognize that we are nothing less than pure awareness.

I am suggesting not that the experience of our individual nature utterly disappears but that it no longer occupies the forefront of our awareness. As we bring the totality of our being into balance, it stills itself. We come to a profound insight into the foundation of our individuality. This has a lasting impact on our awareness of the field of our experience, as we recognize that self and Self are one.

Then personality dissolves. Personality, after all, is like a fog that settles over the land during the night. When the sun comes up in the morning it lifts up the mist and burns it away. So, too, with all personality. When we experience the light of this inner Self, every personality trait becomes unimportant to us, as we realize that we are only one thing. For that matter, when we begin to live from the Self, it is no longer necessary to trace our individual histories. In fact, that history becomes basically irrelevant. What happened when, where, how, why, and to whom ceases to matter to us.

Even though our bodies still exist and our minds and emotions appear to manifest (all of which is natural to the expressive structure of this highest state of energy), we are no longer enmeshed in any of it. Our individual nature simply endures as something like a burr under our saddle for a period of time. We do not escape, deny, or avoid it. What becomes important to us instead is the spirit in which we live our lives and the spirit in which we endeavor.

This is necessary, because our lives can only constitute a caravan of despair if we remain stuck at the level of personality. Basically, life at that level is brutal and unrewarding. Moreover, no change of any real consequence can happen when personality is the point of departure. The universe as a whole is nothing but a constellation of effects. Likewise, our personalities are also a series of effects. If we try to change them in relation to other people, we are only relating as one set of effects to another, or as Rudi would say, from one superficial part of ourselves to another superficial part, and thinking that something deep has happened as a result.

When we pursue real depth, however, we discover that alterations in the aspect of consciousness from which we are operating give rise to different forms of experience. In one form we perceive an external world that is alive; in another our own interior world predominates. Then there is a third world in which neither of the two appears as distinct and in which there is no apparent cognition whatsoever. How can there be cognition as we know it when the notions of subject and object cease to be meaningful?

I sometimes have the feeling that people think of transcending our individuality and our personalities as a loss or as some sort of ultimate disappointment or emptiness. For that reason, they find it frightening. Yet it is not like that. The denial or, if you will, the negation of our limited awareness leads us instead to the experience of unity and oneness, of Life as an unbounded, infinite whole.

It is like making love with somebody whom you care about deeply: You disappear, the other person disappears; indeed, all experience of separation between the two of you dissolves, and there is only one thing happening. The same thing is true of going beyond the finitude of our humanity. Therefore, transcending our individuated awareness involves no pessimism whatsoever. In fact, it is a wonderful thing to recognize the true reality of our existence. It is like something that has been on the fringes of our awareness during all those moments in our lives when we felt there was something more that we were somehow not managing to get at.

To understand this changes the whole way in which our minds function. It changes what we look for in relationships, what we expect in the world, and what we hope for from ourselves. We see how much this contact with the Self diminishes the importance of material things and of recognition in any superficial, egotistical sense.

Moreover, our minds and emotions are no longer influenced in rigid, limited ways by our biology. We appreciate the reach and range of feeling that manifests within us and allow it to find its appropriate mode of expression in our field of experience. A certain emotional and intellectual richness, as well as an extended and diverse capacity for beauty, manifest themselves in our lives even at the simplest levels. We discover fulfillment within ourselves, even as we recognize who "I" is and always was.

At that stage we know ourselves to be even more than one with God. Why do I put it in these terms? If I were to say that we recognize ourselves to be one with God, that would imply some sort of original separation that has now been resolved. We cannot say this, however, because the real recognition is that there never was anything else but our own total identity with the supreme in the first place.

Truth of this kind is impossible to wrap our minds around. Only when we stop our minds, calm our emotions, and become quiet can we appreciate the infinite, creative process that we are. Only when we are still do we see the infinity within the infinite. When we examine this carefully, we begin to understand the assertion that the highest state is consciousness. We refine our understanding of that, and live in constant communion with that highest awareness of our own awareness.

Awareness of the Self

We have talked about shaktopaya as an awareness of the energy of Life Itself, or of spanda. Yet, even with this awareness of all things and all events as a flow and exchange of energy, we still also operate with the awareness of the distinctions between things. This is why anavopaya is sometimes referred to as the awareness of diversity (*bheda*), and shaktopaya as the awareness of unity in diversity (*bhedabheda*).

Gradually, however, even this sense of diversity begins to dissolve as our awareness becomes more and more established in the experience of all things as expressions of one, infinite energy. This awareness is referred to as shambhavopaya, or awareness of the Self. (We could just as easily call it the awareness of our awareness.) It takes us almost completely beyond all sense of differentiation, and establishes us in the understanding that there is nothing that is not the Self, nothing that is not the same, fundamental energy of spanda. This is referred to as *abheda* ("without differentiation").

In the following chapters, we will talk about this quality of awareness by continuing the discussion of the three fundamental elements of our practice: teacher, meditation, and extending our creative energy. This time though, we will do so from the perspective of shambhavopaya. So we will talk about the Self teaching the Self, we will look at how shamb- havopaya is the strategy that has no strategy, and we will talk about total surrender, or the awareness of the Self. Finally, we will see how these things comes together in the discussion of *mahavyapti*, or "universal integration." This is shambhavopaya, the strategy of Shiva.

The Strategy of the Self

THE SELF AS TEACHER

*The Self is the primary guru, the secondary guru is the
one who initiates. To do and to teach is the secondary
guru, to realize is the primary . . . The secondary guru
leads you to the well. The primary guru drinks from it.*

— NITYANANDA

The Self Teaching Itself

One of the foundation texts of Kashmir Shaivism, the
Pratyabhijnahrdyam, says that the philosophy of Kashmir Shaivism is like a single spoke of a wheel. All philosophies and spiritual traditions are such spokes, extending from the highest
reality. They radiate forth from that highest reality, and yet no
single one of them can encompass it as a whole. Shaivism,
therefore, addresses on the front side the mind's inability to
grasp the ultimate. To go beyond this limitation, it presents a
body of techniques and methods with which to train and
direct our attention to the heart of Life Itself so that *it* may
teach us about itself.

Different texts talk about the search for God, truth, or
something of the kind. At a deeper level of discussion, however,

261

since there is only one thing that we are part of, and that is also a part of us, we are not really searching for anything at all. If there *is* a search, it is for understanding. We hope to have mental and emotional clarity grow within us, along with our understanding of the nature of our bodies, our mental and emotional mechanisms, and their foundation.

As we have seen, in the beginning we talk about a person's practice as creative energy that flows from one place to another. This is somewhat like opening the door and giving a person an elementary-school manual on how a nuclear reactor works. "Put a rod in here, and that thing in there, and you'll have yourself an event." It is much more sophisticated than that, but still we must start out by noticing the this-and-that.

Later we become aware of everything as energy, and as a vast process of exchange. At some stage, however, there has to be a quantum leap in our awareness, where we enter into a sustained, direct awareness of the highest reality Itself. Some moment must happen that stills the mind powerfully and engages us deeply enough that this whole experience and understanding can come forth. The question is, who teaches this to us?

The conscious energy of Life Itself is purely Self-expressive, and the universe is the manifestation of its expressive capability. This is another way of saying that consciousness is also self-liberating. What does this mean? We have seen in the discussion of spanda that pulsation is intrinsic to the nature of the highest reality. As it manifests, it conceals the fullness of its nature. Likewise, it also works to disclose that same fullness. In this way it is self-liberating. Of course, only from our individualized point of view is this so. From the perspective of the absolute, this is the same thing as saying that Life Itself is Self-expressive.

This impulse toward liberation comes from the Self and exists in all of us. It is the longing we feel to know something deeper within ourselves. This being so, it is difficult to explain why some people thirst after spiritual knowledge while most people are not interested in the slightest. It remains a paradox.

The point is that all paradoxes resolve in an infinity. Indeed, that is the only place they *can* resolve.

Nevertheless, this does not change the reality that we are all part of that greater creative expression whether we feel moved to know it or not. Everything is this one reality recognizing itself, teaching itself *about* itself over and over again. In our own experience it is a mysterious process that happens by grace.

Because of what the ancient Indian philosophers describe as the ubiquitousness of consciousness, we human beings have the capacity to reflect on our own nature in ways that other organisms do not appear to be capable of. These thinkers would say that our self-examining capacity is intrinsic not only to being human but to the very being of infinite consciousness. It is a demonstration of the universal Self-disclosure and release, in which the Self teaches the self that the two are one and the same.

The Energy of Life Does Everything

One caveat, however. To say that the individualized self and the infinite Self are one and the same can give rise to the possibility for some confusion in how we talk about God. For example, we may slide back and forth between the first and second person, not quite sure whether we should be talking about an "I" or a "you." For that matter, there has been all sorts of fuss at one point or another about whether God is a he, a she, or an it.

Each of these alternatives contains the potential for misunderstanding. If God is the "I" we are talking about, then we could be suggesting that the world of *my* personal sensory experience and what that world feels like to *me* is all there is. Moreover, if it is *me*, then *my* effort should be to transform my universe, and the capacity to transform my universe should be a demonstration of *my* power.

That idea can break down pretty quickly into an inflated understanding of the individualized self. Indeed, one of the objections of the dualists to the nondualists has long been that there is a certain arrogance in saying that we are not separate from the divine. The nondualists respond by saying, "Yes, there is that risk, but that doesn't change how things are. For that matter, show us a real example of something that is truly *other*."

The nondualists go on to suggest other counterarguments, too. For example, the difficulty with buying into the notion of God as some "other" is that we are then not exactly responsible for our own conduct. We have this other to propitiate who may be just as fickle and screwy as we are. That, indeed, is cause for concern. Furthermore, it generates the idea that we should somehow be able to work out some kind of a deal. There should be some angle we can take out on it. Both situations lead us to think we can plan, or at least structure, our life experience.

How does this play itself out in ways that can keep us from learning what the inner teacher is trying to show us? One big way is that we view ourselves as having power, an opinion we base on our daily experience. It is easy to pick up a cup, move it to a different place on the table, and expect it to stay where we put it. From there it is not all that big a jump to the belief that our lives are about *doing* things and making them happen the way we want them to.

After all, when we have a problem we usually want to *do* something rather than let go of the situation. It usually seems easier to compress than to release. Nor is this just true of people in our day and age. The philosophical part of Abhinavagupta's great synthesis of Kashmir Shaivism, the *Tantraloka*, involves a discussion of how, because of their limited perspective, people get caught up in the notion that there is a world in which they exist to *do* something.

This linear logic of cause-and-effect gives us the idea that we have some control over our lives, at least within our own limited band of time and space. We don't usually stop and think that there are many such bands of time and space, from the subatomic level to that of the planets and further out, all of which play some part in our experience. At those broader levels we are in another dimension of the divine, one where we don't have the same kind of power to move things around and put them where we want them.

At the same time, we usually don't recognize the farthest-reaching outcomes of our actions and how they have a ripple effect that extends way beyond our immediate circumstances. For the most part, we don't have to because we are able to sustain our limited notions of power by being able to move things around a little. This approach to power and action usually finds its way into our spiritual work as well. This can become a big problem because, as we saw in the discussion of siddhis, we suddenly find ourselves thinking, "*I* did this," instead of saying, "Oh — the same power that expresses *me* did *this*!" It is a case of getting mixed up about what "I" means. Also, it shows that where we start from shapes where we get to. Duality only engenders more duality.

What I am working around to is that no effort made from an individual perspective can bring about our awakening. Whether we identify the infinite power by which we function as our own or as some other, there is no effort we can make to control the unfolding of our awareness.

We don't always take well to this idea. For the most part, people have small minds, tiny understandings, and are riddled with arrogance and egotism. (And these are the good things we can say.) Moreover, when we are absorbed in our individuality, we constantly restructure every kind of feedback into that perspective. This gives way in time; but then, there is no condition that does not give way in time, even if it takes our dying to do it.

The recognition of shambhavopaya is that it is the energy of Life Itself that does everything, without exception. This is why Rudi used to talk about the nothingness of human beings and the everythingness of God. Everything we experience is the divine concealing and disclosing itself. It is my own feeling that the spirit has the potential to do whatever it wills, at any point in time. I am not exactly a religious person, but still I say it is really God that does everything. We do nothing. In fact, it is hard to accept just how much nothing we do.

Ironically, what we try to *do* to bring about our own vision of how we think things should go only becomes a matter of stepping on our own feet. When we approach our lives in this way, we create problems and tensions that have nothing to do with our reality but only with our illusions. This is true in every aspect of our lives. Our spiritual work is no exception.

The discriminating person whose awareness has been refined through practice learns to recognize and rely on the divine will. He or she does not confuse it with our endlessly changing kaleidoscope of personal desires and ambitions. There is the recognition that what happens in our lives is nothing but a manifestation of this spirit and what it teaches us. The person who is confused about this is the one who only continues to rebuild the illusions that deny his or her access to the true inner potential.

For that matter, the term "potential" is subject to great misunderstanding. It has nothing to do with the potential to *do* anything; indeed, our potential is different. It does nothing and in no way responds to our individual wills. Why do I say that everything that happens in our lives does so from the creative energy out of which everything emerges? Because this energy has its own dynamic and momentum.

This means we can have a long wish list of what we think we want in our lives, and basically, it doesn't do us a bit of good. We may even say to ourselves, "I'm making a personal decision to go out and get this thing or that." Then we do so and fall flat on our faces. Even when we *make* the thing happen, we find we didn't really get what we wanted. Why? Because we decided to do something that the energy was not really allowing to take place.

Of course, we can try to force the issue. But then, we have to understand that if we play in the traffic enough, Life, like any real teacher, probably figures we *want* to play in the traffic, and lets us do so. Therefore, we should not feel too bad when we get hit by a car, since essentially it is what we asked for.

If there is anything at all that our lives are trying to teach us, it is this: Any action not done from total surrender to the recognition that the energy of Life Itself does everything is done out of fear and insecurity. Invariably such actions result in tensions and give rise to manipulation. Anything having the substance and potential for real change originates only from the energy. Then it seems as though things simply happen, with nothing forcing them at all. This is action done from a state of surrender.

As beginners, we *do* things. As advanced people, we don't *do* anything. We simply observe and experience the natural vitality of our own essence. We then have the opportunity to develop an intuitive sense of the dynamics of Life Itself. As we learn to step back and take an increasingly integrated view of our lives, we see that these dynamics are so big that there is nothing we can do except surrender. Our attempts to change things only set up circumstances that are even messier and that we will also have to surrender.

This tells us that our task in life is to surrender and allow Life Itself to be the teacher. Our qualities, gifts, and talents are independent of anything we have or do. They find ways to work themselves out in the world, but only grace really does anything. We could just as easily say that love does everything.

I have always trusted in that love. It is what teaches us about the real nature of Life. It has never failed me; indeed, I have never seen it fail anybody. Furthermore, we discover that when we live in a deep state of surrender, established in what Nityananda called *vira vairagya*, or "the heroic state of non-attachment," then the energy often does what we ask, but in a more sophisticated way. Because we have peeled away our sense of limited identity, the unity we establish within the depth of ourselves merges our will with the divine will, the self into the Self.

At the highest level of our practice, there is no longer any *doing* as we are used to thinking of it. Certainly, there is no thought or wish for anything. There is, however, the proper posture: a relaxed physical body, the awareness of every single breath, and a profound openness that is possible only from a state of complete surrender.

Then we experience something fine and deep coming out of us. We can call it the Self loving the Self, God's love or grace, or consciousness teaching itself. All of these are the same thing.

Free Will

When I say that, being self-liberating, the energy teaches us about itself, people sometimes wonder where the notion of free will fits into the discussion. On one level this is a question asked by the ego, which wants to know if it is giving up the right to have opinions about anything ever again for as long as it lives. On another level, however, free will is a way of talking about our freedom to make choices in the context of a much larger process.

This is an important point because everything we do, without exception, is the outcome of real choices that we make. These choices may rarely demonstrate much awareness of the big picture, but they are still real. Even when we are in circumstances that completely confine our range of possibility, we still make the choice of the attitude with which we will respond. This choice we always have.

Whatever choice we make, that choice becomes a dynamic event that we have loosed and for which we are responsible. Once we are on the pony, we are on the pony. If it is friskier than we thought, we had better hold on or find a soft spot to land. So when we make a choice, whether knowingly or unknowingly, how we respond to its unfolding is up to us. The issue it is not so much a question of the circumstances in which we find ourselves but of how we deal with them. This is like Rudi's story of the mouse that finds itself trapped in a 500 pound bag of flour. Does it freak out and suffocate, or patiently begin to eat its way out? In a case like that, freaking out might not be the best choice.

Nor is it a matter of making informed choices. If we live in a state of complete surrender, to talk of "informed choices" is not necessary. The awakening of our insight and intuitive faculties allows us to make decisions that are informed by something much deeper than any concrete data or information. They are based, instead, on the ability to look at a small section of a dynamic event and, from that, to have some sense of the trajectory it is taking.

From there we think about whether or not that is where we want to go. Is this a field in which we want to be planted? In one sense, it doesn't really matter in what field we are planted, since, ultimately, all of them are Potters' Field. When we realize that every field is ultimately a graveyard, we don't get planted there in the first place.

We are always free. This is not only our condition now; it was our condition yesterday, the day before yesterday, last year, and five years ago. It will remain the same forever. Only our imprisonment in the stream of experience causes us not to recognize this fundamental condition. Yet until we can begin to imagine this possibility, how will we experience it or have the conviction that it is real?

In a sense, Life lived deeply teaches us that there are no wrong choices. Any choice can cut both ways. To a great degree, it depends on a person's attitude as to whether something is a pure or impure event. The texts say that, on one level, those things closer to consciousness are pure, while those that are not so close are impure. Yet, since everything is consciousness in the first place, the notion that impurity exists is ultimately questionable.

I observe that people will usually be energized by their practice to go and do one thing or another. The problem with *doing* is that it is difficult to overcome that momentum and enter a state of nondoing. Once we enter that state of doing, few people can release into nondoing.

Still, there is always the choice. The scope, compassion, depth of feeling, largeness of vision, and sophistication of intelligence available to a human being is the highest reality shining through us. If we can take all our experience and convert it into this profound understanding, then we have grown immensely from it. Given the few choices we do have, certainly we can pick something better than we often do.

Being people committed to living heroic lives compels us to search for and engage in those choices, just as it calls us to manifest them.

If our loving can affect the world in some simple way, it is not because we will build great cities or even do anything anywhere outside ourselves. It is because we open our hearts, embrace the truth within ourselves, trust it, allow it to teach us, and live steadfastly in the awareness of that truth, demonstrating it in our lives with others. This is the real choice we have every day. When we can do this, we can truly say we have freed ourselves: We have met the Teacher, and it is us.

THE MEANS THAT ARE NO MEANS

Give up honor and pride, give up love of body. Only then can you see God everywhere and in every being.

— NITYANANDA

Not By Any Means

Shambhavopaya is not an upaya in the usual sense of the word, because "upaya" generally refers to a vehicle or a strategy and implies some kind of an effort. Shambhavopaya, however, is not an effort. There is no question of exertion of any kind. Nor is it something that can be proved by logical means, because all means of proof owe their existence to it and cannot be used to prove their own source. So it cannot be arrived at through any vikalpa, or thought construct, but only in a state in which all reasoning has dissolved into the conviction that the self and the Self are one and the same.

For that matter, Abhinavagupta also says that this awareness does not come to us as a result of meditation; Shiva, he says, never reveals himself through meditation. This has to be so, because any method, itself, comes by grace. Unlike anavopaya, it is not responsive to efforts of our will. So shambhavopaya is a yoga for which no process of our minds or our breath can accomplish anything. Rather, shambhavopaya means the *bhav*, the "perspective," or "view," of Shiva, one of whose names is Shambhu. Therefore Shambhavopaya is the God's-eye view of reality. It is the means for which there are no means.

This makes it, in one sense, the simplest of all the upayas because it requires no effort or discipline. On the other hand, it is the most subtle and difficult because we are so used to trying to get at things through some kind of exertion. When we try to get free of the vikalpas, for example, we usually only end up setting up new vikalpas. It is sort of like trying to jump out of our own skins.

It is better to think of shambhavopaya not as something we achieve, but as something we unwrap, or unveil. We cannot *make* the vikalpas go away, but we can release all effort to hold on to them. Abhinavagupta says that when we are able neither to accept nor reject a vikalpa, it will retire of itself and we will find ourselves to be what we are. This is why the awareness of shambhavopaya is sometimes called an artless art. It is spontaneous, without effort. Sometimes it comes about by an awakening imparted by the guru through shaktipat; sometimes we experience an unexpected, intensive awakening through some other circumstance usually thought of as an expression of grace. In any case, it is something over which we have absolutely no control whatsoever.

You might think that if this awareness has nothing to do with any proof or method — that if upaya means strategy, and I am telling you there *is* no strategy — then how is it possible? Doesn't that make it unknowable? The question is reasonable, but this is not what the Trika masters were saying at all. Instead, they were talking about an awareness that comes to us on its own, in a spontaneous flash. This, they said, was the shortest path. It is a conscious moment during which something breaks in on our awareness and discloses the divine.

They tried to suggest different kinds of moments when this could happen, by referring to ordinary experiences we have all had. Think, for example, of the intense delight you feel when you see a beloved friend or relative after a long absence, or of the feeling you have when you hear news that makes you either extremely happy or disappointed. Think about the amazement you feel when you suddenly see something you have never seen before, the strong fear you feel in the face of something terrifying; think of some moment of pure fury. It can be the beginning or end of a sneeze or of hunger. It can be the vertigo of hanging over the edge of a cliff, when you can neither go forward nor climb to safety. It is the moment of greatest intensity of all these states. What each of them has in common is this intensity.

When any one of these conditions is strained to its limit in a moment of extreme intensity, it is as though we *are* nothing but our delight or fear, our vertigo or our anger, our hunger or even our sneeze. It is in moments of concentration such as these that the mind comes to a dead stop. All our other mental activities cease by themselves in a moment of instant shock that throws us into the very core, or heart, of our being.

This is not brought about by meditation; we practice meditation as a way of quieting all the ways our minds get restless. Meditation is also the way we orient our wills toward knowing this deepest reality. It is the way we concentrate our entire being on becoming aware of our own deepest awareness. It is these kinds of intense experiences, however, that bring the mind to a halt. Then, in the midst of this simple awareness, free of all conceptualization, a spontaneous flash of insight comes to us. It is direct and immediate. For me, it happened when I met Rudi.

It is as though our awareness leaps beyond itself into an instantaneous, intuitive understanding. It cuts through everything in a flash and changes forever how we see the world. It absorbs us into a field of love. I could also say that such a jolt throws us right into direct contact with spanda, the vibration of our inner reality. It gives us the immediate experience of spanda and, therefore, of the very source of our being.

We recognize this if we are alert to it. This is the point of our regular practice. The practice itself is not what makes anything happen, but it is what has quieted our minds enough that we are able to know it when we see it and to sustain our awareness of it. If we are wide awake we hold on to it. If we are not, the moment simply passes us by. It is said that then we remain stupefied and bewildered.

Think about all the times you have been in the grip of some intense emotion and gotten choked by it. There is no guarantee that we will know in that moment to turn our attention inside. In fact, most of the time we don't. Instead, we get lost in the delight, the fear, or the anger, instead of going to their source.

On the other hand, when we are able to get to the heart of the matter, this is awakening. At the same time, it is not "liberation" or "enlightenment" in the way people often think of these things. We do not acquire some new condition.

Rather we simply come back to the awareness of the freedom we can never lose. It is not a new consciousness but the awakening of the consciousness that was always there.

This is the direct apprehension of the highest reality. It is the mental condition and outlook of a person who experiences the highest state of self-awareness, a person dissolved in the divine. As this state emerges and we experience the profound conviction that necessarily arises from it, our whole understanding and our total pattern are transformed forever.

In this experience, all the techniques we have studied come together in a single, undifferentiated intuition — the one means that is no means at all. This phase cannot be sought after. That is why it is said that it emerges by grace. We cannot learn it or work to attain it. The only thing we can do is surrender.

Total Surrender

The *Maharthamanjari* says, "All that one can surrender, surrender it, without question. It is this which one must reject. That which one absolutely cannot surrender, it is this which must be acquired. The Self, immutable by nature, is the only thing we cannot shed." All the work we do to release our blocks and tensions and to create a greater flow within and around ourselves is simply a preparatory stage for entering into the reality of the one thing we cannot shed: the dynamic stillness at the center of ourselves. We intensify that flow within us and observe the ways in which we extend it, even as we begin to experience and understand that it is the essence of every flow.

Earlier, I said that this refinement of our practice begins with a total commitment to growing. As we cultivate our awareness we discover that this statement is both true and not true. It is true in the sense that we must gather up our many scattered desires into a clear focus on growing. In this way our energy and effort take on a unified orientation, regardless of the diversity of our activities.

The statement is not true, however, in the sense that advanced practice goes beyond any kind of commitment.

Indeed, at this stage the very notion of commitment, insofar as it suggests the imposition of our will on a situation, comes to seem like a certain arrogance. No commitment can bring us to the point of surrender that is the essence of advanced practice. As we realize that the power of spirit does everything and we do nothing, the idea that we make anything happen at all through our will becomes the potential source for tremendous misunderstanding. This we saw in the discussion of siddhis.

Initially we develop a commitment because we discover something that functions in our interest and figure that it makes sense to pursue it. This is not a bad thing, but it represents a limited take on the situation. If we want to know the highest reality as an object, we can only fail, because it can never be reduced to an object. We are still seeking some benefit and therefore thinking in terms of gain and loss.

The ultimate attainment is already ours, but the experience of it comes to us only when we are in a state of complete surrender. In this case, "surrender" means the surrender of everything — every effort, desire, thought of attainment or, indeed, anything that represents the thought of any *other* — as we become centered, instead. The person who is able to do this becomes a fountain of consciousness.

But to get to *that*, we have to give up all this; and when we don't know what *that* is, it is a difficult thing to do. Ordinarily, people would rather endure a terrible situation with which they are familiar than take on something wonderful with which they are not. The transition, for most people, is unendurable. Yet as our individuality dissolves, and as we come more and more into contact with the increasingly abstract and refined aspects of our existence, what we think of as our wants and needs begin to look pretty puny.

This capacity for surrender is not a matter of conceptual understanding. Nor is it based on the mastery of texts. Rudi, for example, never studied any texts. During the last year or so of his life, however, he was formulating what he called his Tantric work. This Tantric work he put together from the depth of his own psyche. In retrospect, however, it looks much as though he was rewriting the *Shiva Sutras* from the heart of his experience. The mechanisms he lays out are those described in the discussion of the upayas. This is why it was exciting for me to encounter Kashmir Shaivism and the *Shiva Sutras*. It was also encouraging because I saw a continuity of practice and experience carried through in my own lineage, even as it coincided with an event that was much older.

The character of Rudi's Tantric work differs from the earlier work he gives, which is more in keeping with themes we have already discussed. Rudi emphasized working, devotion, and commitment — essentially, breaking oneself into little pieces. His was the marine corps of spiritual practices, although the marine corps is probably a little easier because they let a person off occasionally. At Rudi's, we were on twenty-four hours a day, seven days a week, every week, month in and month out.

Rudi's practice was this: You deeply want to grow with your whole heart and soul. All the mechanisms of the practice aim at acquiring that deep, intense feeling. As that yearning to grow matures, it becomes a profound love of God and a deep passion for Life. This passion is not directed toward the objects of the material world but toward knowing, in the deepest sense, the vitality that animates everything.

Rudi described the transition from this regular practice to his Tantric work as the surrender of *everything*. At a certain point we recognize that even growing is no longer the issue. We notice a shift from wanting to grow, to sensing the need to release our attachment to everything. This is what Rudi talked about as complete surrender.

Even the desire to be without goal or purpose, without need or desire, is a tension. This is because every desire is essentially the same thing. At a certain point, because of the existence of what we might call grace, or because of our careful study of the situation over time, we begin to recognize that any desire, however noble, is an obstruction to the fulfillment of our search. Even this desire signifies that we are not truly free of conceptualizing. In a way, the desire to liberate ourselves is the one remaining obstacle we face. This orientation only begins to break down as the flow we awaken within ourselves not only revitalizes our lives on one level but, on another level, transcends our lives as we know them.

Rudi said that even when we want to surrender and try to do so, we rarely understand that this means total surrender. Usually there is some area in which we feel we do not have to surrender or in which we can wait. But if our surrender is to be authentic, we must let go of everything. He observed that, after all, tying a rope around yourself and letting yourself down the side of the mountain is not the same as jumping off and falling into space.

We can decide to change our orientation in this way at any point in time. Of course, if we are wrong in our timing, we will confuse this decision with not needing to do any further inner work. Then we will suffer a backlash that will kick our teeth in. If nothing else, this will be exciting and dramatic, although it may well have dire consequences for our lifelong investment in spiritual work.

As Rudi made the shift from the regular work into his Tantric work, he said, "We no longer ask to grow spiritually, but to surrender everything." He expressed this in a brief prayer, in which he said, "I surrender all things: thought, form, matter, sound, everything." That prayer was his stepping stone between the highest level of the *Shiva Sutras* and the teaching he was giving me at the time of his death.

Moments before the plane crash that was to kill him, Rudi recorded these words:

"I feel the last year of my life has prepared me for the understanding that expanded consciousness can only come through expanded nothingness. This state is produced by surrendering the tensions that bind and restrict our physical mechanism from expressing the power of creation. It is God flowing through us and showing us how we are connected to Him as the expression of higher creative will and a deeper sense of surrender."

The paradox is that when we enter into the state of total surrender, we discover that we have actually given up nothing at all. We have surrendered the self into the Self, the finite consciousness into the unlimited. It is like throwing a match into a forest fire, surrendering fire into fire.

How is it possible to let go of our lives completely in this way? We just do it. Actually, it is this simple: As long as there is no fuel, there can be no fire; as long as there is fuel, we burn on. All I can tell you about it is that it is not so difficult to burn away the tensions of our individual lives when our attention is centered on fusing with and in the infinite. Then we sustain our individual, everyday lives, bringing them to material, emotional, and mental equilibrium, even as we stay centered in the midst of the fire.

Finally the sense of purpose that drives us dissipates. If there is only one highest reality, then we have no purpose beyond *its* purpose, which is nothing but the joyous articulation of its own creative content. This is not what we usually think of as purpose, so it changes our whole point of view and our whole situation. What I am getting at is related to the joy of doing, itself, that is implicit in the structure of all manifestation.

Like nonattachment, purposeless awareness is not something to which we can actively aspire. Rather it is a state we enter because we are vigilant and connected to the flow of energy within and around us. That pure state is purposeless. It is, as the Tibetan Buddhist teacher Trungpa Rinpoche once called it, "the journey without goals." Having no differentiation, judgment, or distinction, it is that pure, vital awareness, the witness of its own drama as it unfolds.

When we arrive in that state of purposeless awareness, we simply relax and enjoy it. We are not nervous about the fact that there is nothing to be done, no place to go, and no further effort to make. These things do not agitate us or cause us to think that perhaps we are doing something wrong. Instead, we understand that true spiritual growth is free from purpose, mission, and destiny. It requires the strength to transcend the seduction of everything worldly and the recognition that our sole support is God. There is, after all, no other.

Anavopaya encompasses action and thought pointed toward a goal, which is to grow. It takes our scattered efforts and unfocused will and, in their place, cultivates a sense of purpose, a will directed toward an end to be realized. It cannot avoid the duality of thinker and thought. Still, it is useful because it unfolds into the awareness of shaktopaya and even, with grace, into the awakening of shambhavopaya. In all of this, surrender is the key.

THE AWARENESS OF THE SELF

To grow spiritually is to see everything as God.

— RUDI

Living Above Our Pain

In the discussion of spanda and the tattvas, it is said that when Shakti turns within, she merges into Shiva and becomes more than herself. The many return into the one. This is the reversing of the process of manifestation. In our experience, this is the transcendence of our individualized identity, the dissolution of separateness and the immersion into our contact with the One.

As this happens we understand that the same energy that gives rise to the whole universe is within us. This is known as realizing the spanda principle. We see that the empirical, psychological complex that we have taken to be ourselves is not at all what we thought it was, and that *this* is our essential Self.

This experience overturns every feeling we have ever had of needing anything. If this is within us — if it *is* us — then how can there be any real absence of anything? We see that most human beings are like people in a lake dying of thirst. We don't see that all the resources we need are within and around us. They are infinite and surpass anything we could ever actually require.

As we enter into continuous contact with the essence of Life Itself, we find that there is no sense of absence, void, or emptiness. We feel no need for anything. It is not necessary to add to what we are or take anything away. There is no issue of improving or getting rid of anything. Rather we experience only the simple recognition of what is.

If it is true that we will never be closer to eternity than we are now, there can be no lack of anything but vision. Discovering that we have enough, that nothing is missing, and that our lives are a wonder, how can we not be completely at peace? Basically we understand in the profoundest way that Life Itself has no problems.

This means that the fundamental core of our lives is without issues. Therefore the very notion of problems, needs, desire, and external accumulation is a misunderstanding — a fraud, if you will — that our biology has perpetrated upon us. This awareness brings about a relaxation in our bodies, a quiet to our minds, a joyousness to our hearts, and a fullness all around us that is extraordinary. How even to describe it? That is the difficult part.

When we understand the ephemeral and superficial nature of the appearances around us, it becomes difficult to get anxious or upset about any of them. No wonder great yogis and spiritual people become nonattached to this world. How can they take it all that seriously? They know that if you stick around for another two minutes, the whole situation changes. This being so, what is there to get excited about or chase after? Why get stuck in repeating the mantra of stupidity?

As we experience the consciousness at the core of our existence, the suffering we assume to be a necessary part of our lives is also alleviated. We may feel pain, but we no longer suffer. We may feel all the experiences that affect our bodies and persist in our ordinary lives, but they neither limit nor bring us down. Instead, we see in the form of every feeling and action the presence of the divine. We feel that infinite potentiality within ourselves at each and every moment.

Nityananda's greatness as a spiritual being did not, in any way, relieve him from the painful arthritis he endured for a long time. By the end of his life he could not bend his knees, elbows, or fingers and he had a great deal of pain in his back. He also had a liver disorder that resulted in the constant distension of his belly.

One might ask why he didn't heal himself. It may have been that although he did heal other people, he subsequently paid for it himself. The tension, after all, has to go some place; it doesn't just evaporate. Either that, or he was so unattached to material circumstances that he simply didn't care. He himself felt that the energy was not to be used for one's own benefit, even when this meant one lived with constant pain.

Here is evidence that this state does not remove the structural issues from our lives. (Structural issues are all the things we have to face in the circumstances of our lives.) One example of this for me was Rudi's passing. All the awareness and fulfillment in the universe could not help me avoid that experience or any of the others that followed it.

At a certain point, however, we find that such experiences themselves are not the issue. We still experience disappointments and pain, as well as a great deal of joy. The difference is that none of it, neither the pain nor the joy, disturbs our equilibrium. Even the painful situations in our lives take place as part of a total event, one that continuously reorganizes what we are and further develops our potential for self-expression.

This is possible because the ordinary consciousness of the individual is relational; it is always based on some sense of subject and object, some duality. Pleasure comes from our attraction to something other; pain is caused by our tension with that other. Always our psychological states are conditioned by this assumption of relationship. But in the awareness of the highest state a person is free of the duality of subject and object. So the causes of pleasure and pain are absent. Even when these experiences occur, they do not affect such a person, because he or she sees everything only as an expression of the delight of spanda.

Rudi was like this. He used to talk about the paintings of Tibetan beings dancing above fire as being similar to his own state. "I lived above my pain," he said. "I was so busy reaching beyond the level of my particular agony that I did not sink into it. A child could remove me from this depth of despair for half a day. The scent of a flower gave me twenty minutes of peace. I have gotten high as a kite over a new pair of socks. The ability to love everything saved me. I found the narcotic of life enabled me to transcend the pain of existence. Everything and anything became essential for me. It taught me to appreciate all things." This kind of suffering is no suffering.

I said earlier that even painful situations develop our potential for self-expression. When I say "self-expression," I am not talking about finger-painting. Rather I am talking about the expression of the Self, the vital, creative power that revitalizes and renews us at all times. The symphony of Life unfolding from within us is an entirely beneficial event. Its sole purpose, if we can even speak in such terms, is to free us. When we understand this, we see that there is never a reason to feel any real fear. We become, in other words, free from fear. In this state we find the strength, peace, and clarity to face whatever we must, every single day. This is both our innermost resource and something that extends infinitely beyond us.

Indeed, we become free to express our lives in a continuously positive and constructive way. We have no need to become entangled in things, to become angry or bitter. Nor do we feel any need for recrimination. We don't allow the tensions of our lives to freeze our muscles, rot our bodies, or limit our biology and chemistry to expressing themselves in rigid and structured ways. Because we discover the infinite resource, the very essence of our own lives, we have no further need to compete with others, to become angry, or to experience greed or jealousy.

So we don't respond to violence with violence, because we understand the vicious cycle that this represents. We see how the potential for good is consumed and destroyed in useless competition and a vicious cycle of violent interaction. Because we find fulfillment inside, we become free from the violence and struggle that arise from the perception of lack and absence.

Even when we find ourselves initially confused in a situation, we never have to stay deluded or confused by all of the different atmospheric changes we encounter. We have an inner frame of reference that provides us with understanding and continuity. That simple frame of reference is the experience of total well-being implicit in the contact with our inner Self.

The essence of Life Itself is one simple dynamic that is by nature balanced and harmonious. At the same time, it also manifests as a broad field of action in which many different pressures and tensions, and many different levels of density, are formed. As we move in this broader medium of conscious energy, its various densities and pressures have an effect on our minds and emotions. As we become able to tune into the subtlest level on which all phenomena exist, however, we are never thrown off balance.

If we do get out of sync with the highest state we will know it because something will hit us in the nose. Suddenly there will be the appearance of an *other*, and the manifestation of tension. Then our nose will get out of joint, which will inform us immediately that we are not in the highest state. Why? Because in the highest state, there is nothing there to punch me in the nose; there is only myself.

Fortunately, however, we are grounded in an understanding of who and what we are, why we are here, and what it is all about. That frees us from the roller coaster, the microperspective of the nonsensical that happens on a daily basis. It allows us to rise above the petty tensions in which people get enmeshed every day and frees us to live in a state of creative flow and conscious capability. Then a profound, dynamic serenity permeates all our experience with the joy of the highest Presence, in which nothing is absent.

Total Freedom

We say that consciousness is free and unbounded in every way, but what does this mean? "Freedom" is one of those tricky words, a little bit like "love." It is hard to say just what it means, because there are so many different definitions. Of course, consciousness is difficult to talk about in general because, as we have seen in the discussion of matrika, words are only implicit in consciousness. They become an expression of it, but not vice versa. This means that there are no words capable of encompassing and fully articulating it.

Words can only lead us along the path of contemplation. In order to grasp what lies behind them, we have to practice and experience it ourselves in order to understand what these teachers were attempting to communicate through the different sutras. Still, what we can say about it is that this absolute consciousness is infinitely free and unbounded in every way. In its infinite freedom it is both infinitely creative and infinitely joyful. At the same time this free will is the very heart of the divine.

The basic power of the ultimate reality is called *svatantrya*, or total freedom. This freedom has two aspects. One is that it exists entirely without external support; it just *is*. The other is that svatantrya also means the freedom to imagine and create without limitation. That is, the energy is completely free to change and evolve. It is not necessarily committed to anything, except to the continuous manifestation of its own power, glory, and vitality.

Since we are individual manifestations of infinite consciousness, each human being is endowed with the same infinite potentiality from which the whole universe has come forth. The state of our inner spirit, the essence of our lives, is at all times, and in every point in time and space, essentially free. If that were not true, then we could not awaken to a deeper awareness. That is, only because that freedom is implicit in our very existence, present now, yesterday, and tomorrow, is the possibility of becoming aware always there. When we recognize the fundamental liberty with which this creative energy endows us, we also recognize that we are free to do whatever we want.

The freedom to change implies the ability to choose or will; it is the capacity to orient our hearts and love. Freedom in and of itself, without will to direct it toward expression, would be meaningless. When we orient the will toward growing, the transformation that takes place within us involves a total revitalization as many of our unpleasant, unfortunate experiences simply get flushed out of the system as a whole.

To recognize the highest self-awareness as the fundamental source of our existence is to incinerate in a flash all our garbage within the fire of that self-awareness. Then instead of living out particular lines of karma — having our lives, minds, and emotions structured by the ways we think we ought to do something or by what we think we didn't do — we are able to look at what is authentic and appropriate to a situation and live from *that* understanding. This is clarity.

From this clarity we see growth taking place on one level, yet we also see that there is no such thing as growth, just as there is no such thing as karma. We enjoy a total freedom in which everything escapes the requirements of logical sequence and of any system of time and causality because we live in the eternal present.

The ever-newness of this highest Self requires that ever-oldness pass away. It requires that there be temporary dimension to all patterns. The Chinese speak of it as "To walk on sand and leave no trace." It is like that. Everything is temporary. This is different, however, from saying that it is untrustworthy. Life is free and doesn't do what we want it to. It doesn't stay the same for long, and it is up to us to reconnect to and participate in it consciously.

We have to rediscover this truth on a regular basis. Otherwise we start to feel out of touch with our environment. So the practice of Trika Yoga, instead of being a process by which a person ascends out of a lived reality to heaven, is one by which we cultivate our awareness of that freedom in life.

The bottom line is that we always have a choice. It may not necessarily be the choice we might like, but no one always gets that. Nevertheless, this becomes irrelevant when we recognize that by engaging and cultivating our free power of choice, something amazing and miraculous happens. Somehow the quality of our lives manages to transcend its own limitations. We find a richness and vibrancy about our lives that is truly wonderful, regardless of how simple or sophisticated our lives may actually be.

Understand that we are completely free and that we have, within ourselves, infinite potentiality. There is nothing to attain. In fact, in this lifetime there is only the exploration of our own universal freedom — a freedom we already have, which is impossible for anything or anyone ever to deny us.

The Creativity of God

Both the vitality of Life and its capacity to create from within itself are what make it divine. Otherwise it would be inert. We have carried on this discussion already. Likewise, creativity is a quality of the divine. In fact, what makes it God *is* creativity. Our human lives are a manifestation of this creativity of God, just as our own creativity is a manifestation of our innate and intimate contact with that highest reality.

We can understand the connection this way: Think about a poem you might write. Is there a difference between the spark of inspiration in which the impulse to write originates and its coalescing into a form that you actually write down as the condensation of that original spark? Is there a distinction between the song to which a person gives voice and the impulse that gives rise to singing in the first place? It begins with a simple introversion, which gives rise to a spark, which gives rise to an impulse, which gives rise to an expression.

What, after all, is a poem if not a feeling that coalesces within us, to which we strive to give words? There is no particular logic that has to be expressed. Rather it is a feeling we attempt to portray, in which the words should support the extension of that feeling. If we cannot keep our attention on that feeling, allowing it to intensify and not escape, we will not have the ability to develop the power of our own creative expression. Whatever we undertake to create most likely begins with some joyous impulse, some small explosion of joy, that goes on to become a manifest project or action.

Since there is no escaping action, and since this creative emission is, in fact, the same as the Self, only the appearance confounds us from recognizing it as such. This is what makes it necessary to understand its source. It is the joy that precedes both the desire for expression, or an expression that may take the form of some desire.

The person who experiences this has a clear, direct, intuitive, and trans-sensory perception of the Self. This is the awareness of oneself as pure consciousness, intimately integrated into the fabric of all of creation.

As a Sword to its Sheath

As long as we have bodies, the issue of surrender persists because the cells keep secreting chemicals to bind us to our environment, just as plants put forth new leaves and tendrils. This, in itself, is not a terrible thing. The only stickiness to it is that if these imperatives do get hold of us, it takes them a long time to let go. Nor does this happen in a flash. Instead, it is like the guests who simply will not go: even when you are ready for them to leave, they don't.

So, everybody has a body and attendant circumstances. As long as we have bodies we will have individual issues of this kind to contend with. They are to be treated like everything else: They are to be surrendered. In this way we avoid being jerked around by their undulations, even as we develop the capacity to extend our awareness of ourselves. There is no other benefit to be experienced from this extension than the deep peace and well-being implicit in the experience of the truth.

Even at this moment, a field of biological imperatives is actively functioning within us. We can never get away from them. We all get hungry, have different urges, and are dimly aware of the chemicals behind them. These, too, are energy because all chemistry has its foundation in energy being transmitted throughout our environment all the time. What we usually don't see is the ways in which the two biological imperatives dominate our existence as powerful and recurring themes. To a great extent they define the horizon of our awareness.

To transcend our humanity is to be in touch with that which is extraordinary about our humanity. It is to put aside that which is common, unintelligent, and brutish about ourselves. Rudi described our physical, material reality as just the tip of the iceberg, as merely one-ninth or one-tenth of our total existence. When we investigate the nature of our own individual reality with some care, we start to understand what we are really all about.

To have this understanding does not free or release us from having to play out our own individual existence. The connection between the highest consciousness and the energy that manifests as biological life, called *prana*, is a natural one. Even though we live from the deepest insight, still our experiences go on and play themselves out in a biological, emotional, and intellectual existence. In other words, just as prana is a natural extension of this highest reality, so is our material existence.

But we understand that our bodies are not what we think they are and, from that, that we are also not what we think we are. As a demonstration of this, we can talk about our bodies, minds, and emotions as a field of experience, interrelated dynamic systems in which the rules of cause and effect apply for only short times and distances. If we recognize this, we can account for many of the disappointing situations in our lives, which are also not what we think they are supposed to be.

When this awareness dawns on us, we are liberated from our earlier suffering, attachments, difficulties, stresses, and strains. In other words, we are liberated from the biological imperatives, which are like a treadmill on which we, as human gerbils, run all day and night. We see, instead, the beauty and the wonder that are the purity of Life Itself.

We become aware of ourselves as luminous beings. Eventually we become so established in this awareness that the discussion of "body" or "not-body" is no longer meaningful. A luminous being doesn't exactly have a body, and the fact that a body is associated with it is more or less incidental. At that point, moreover, it doesn't enter into our awareness to consider the matter in any other way.

A person who recognizes the truth about his or her inner nature still has a body, but he or she is no longer attached to it in any way. At that point the relationship of the spirit to the body is that of a sword to its sheath: While the one might or might not stay in the other, there is no intrinsic connection. Moreover, since the idea of our material bodies is no longer of any importance, we can go in and out of them at will. Indeed, we *do* go in and out at will. This is nothing we make any great effort to do; nor is it a different part of our reality. It just happens.

I don't want to say that we then recognize ourselves to be identical with God, because that is not exactly the case. No matter how profound our awareness becomes, there still remains the element of the biological imperatives. As long as we have bodies, on one level or another we experience being alive as a structured chaos. We might say, though, that as long as he or she has a body the person who experiences shamb-havopaya is *like* Shiva in having many of the characteristics of that highest level of self-awareness. In contrast, after the body is given up, the person is none other than Shiva.

Therefore we don't have the same concern for our own material or physical well-being. The person who has this recognition is a completely free person — free from every kind of problem, limitation, and suffering, free to accept Life as it is and to live with whatever it brings with deep and joy-ous inner peace.

A Sense of Total Well-Being

This freedom, security, and total capability together in one self-awareness, manifest as a feeling often referred to as bliss. I have tried to eliminate this term from my own lan-guage as much as possible, because the word has become cheapened into a cliche that is tossed around in various spiri-tual circles. I prefer, therefore, to speak of a sense of total well-being.

The experience of this is subtle, and it permeates all the different levels of our experience. It refers to the joy that is the motivating event underlying all appearances. Rumi speaks of it as "the secret sky." If you have practiced for a while, you have probably experienced it already and will again. Moreover, it will become clear to you at some stage what is happening. "To fly toward the secret sky" is to experience infinity, to connect to and participate in it.

From various things I had read and heard, I used to imag-ine somehow that the experience of the highest reality would be like the nighttime sky: a vast, open space and a subtle, ethe-real void. Imagine my surprise when, one day as I was following the energy, something broke open and I entered the state of the infinitely full power of Life Itself. It is something like standing in the center of the sun. I discovered that this awakening was not the peace I had heard promoted all along. Rather the fundamental core of our existence is completely full, as it must be. If there is only one thing, then there is only the infinite fullness of infinite awareness, which is completely powerful and infinitely abundant.

This takes us beyond every polarity we have ever encountered: beyond gain and loss, success and failure, or happiness and sadness. For example, there are so many things about which to be happy or sad in this world. But the real issue is not one of being either one or the other. To be in contact with the deepest power of Life Itself is to rise above both and enter into a balanced state of pure awareness, where we appreciate every potentiality. There we find the unbroken experience of total well-being. The point is not one of being either a happy person or a sad one, but of finding fulfillment in our lives.

The union of Shiva and Shakti is a fundamental state of total well-being. Established in this state, which is beyond expansion and contraction, we are simply observers of the expansion and contraction of the universe, the witness of this expression of its creative power. Then we are Shiva who watches Shakti creating but who is never in any way disturbed by that creativity. For Shiva this creativity is entertainment and play carried out for nothing but the joy of it, which is one way of expressing its being without intent or purpose.

Therefore, our existence is one of joy, contentment, and strength. We pass through the different realms of materiality, feeling, and intellect simply and easily, never losing contact with our awareness of the fundamental ground from which we come. In the context of shambhavopaya, there is no real discussion of manifestation. There is no issue of universal process, no talk of energies, no question of form or substance. From the point of view of shambhavopaya, there is nothing but the infinite, spontaneous expression of joy, the essential nature of this highest pure awareness.

This joy has the flavor of complete freedom. Walking in this freedom, we no longer stumble over each of our steps, weighed down by effort. Rather we move freely and easily in the infinite space of total well-being.

Mahavyapti:
The Universal Integration

*When the bliss of consciousness is attained, there is the
lasting acquisition of that state in which consciousness
is our only Self, and in which all things that appear are
identical with consciousness. Even the body that is
experienced appears as identical with the Self.*

— PRATYABHIJNAHRYDAYAM

The awareness of the Self permeates our limited awareness of self in what is called *vyapti*, or "union with the ultimate." This is the finite dissolving into the infinite, extending
itself back out to its expansive unlimitedness. It is a state of
wholeness, stripped of all superficiality, in which there is nothing that is not the Self.

This awareness leads to a total inversion of our senses.
What does this mean? Our senses are completely withdrawn
from their usual state of distraction. Turned within, they rest
in the awareness of the Self. Then all that we experience we
view as nothing but creative energy that is no different from
ourselves.

This doesn't mean that our senses cease to be open to
external objects but that they have come fully under the

influence of the Self. Both our creative resources and our senses, which are the mediators between these resources, are infinite in nature. To recognize this depersonalizes our senses. No longer do we speak of "my vision," because we realize that "my vision" is vision itself. The same holds true for all the senses. So, while they ordinarily serve to keep our attention externalized, in this state the senses act as vehicles that carry us to perceive nothing but the Self.

This becomes true whether we are waking or sleeping. The Trika masters said that there are four states of animation in which we pass our time, the first three of which are waking, dreaming, and deep sleep. The fourth state is the awareness of spanda, the invariable condition that is the background of all we do, even though we are usually unaware of it. Most people sense it, if at all, only at the beginning and end of waking, dream, and deep sleep, and not in the middle of these states. This fourth state the Trika masters called *turya*.

When somehow we emerge into the awareness of shambhavopaya, that awareness sustains itself as turya. It is like something that comes out of hiding to become the active feature of our everyday awareness. Then we have the integral experience of spanda whether we are waking, dreaming, or in deep sleep. Even though these look like different states, there is the glow of an inner light that infuses all of them.

Then we see that the foundational consciousness of Life Itself is not precisely the same as, yet is found within, every state of consciousness with which we walk around and carry on our lives. The highest consciousness is neither separate from, nor to be confused with, these states. Like a thread running through beads, it connects all the others.

Beyond this is the state known as *turyatita*. There a person is immersed in the ocean's depth, beyond ecstasy. He or she perceives no limitation anywhere. Life is integral, and consciousness is eternally active. There is a mutual interpenetration of the total well-being of turya, and that which is beyond it, turyatita. Then a person experiences turya in turyatita, and turyatita in turya.

In this state we think, speak, and act beyond all dualistic thought. What looked at one time like boundaries between things shifts to a process of dynamic interchange. Eventually we see this as the frequencies of oscillation within one reality. This oscillating frequency has finer and finer foundations to it, with increasingly more subtle frequencies.

Having that recognition, we slip into a state of awareness that goes beyond time and space. I say this because the experience of flow, and even of oscillation, is ordinarily related to the experience of temporal and spatial relations. As our awareness expands and becomes more subtle, we become increasingly aware of this subtle dynamic. We recognize that infinity was always there, but that our awareness was contracted around the highly and densely organized manifestation of it that was available to us.

This experience is called samadhi, which refers to being completely absorbed in pure awareness. The *Spandakarikas* speaks of two general kinds of samadhi. One is our experience of ourselves as nothing but the pure vitality of consciousness. This we experience with our eyes closed as we meditate to free ourselves from the limitations we imagine we are. We relax, forget about our bodies, and quiet our minds. In this way we attune ourselves to the simple vitality that permeates our entire existence. That vitality is not separate from our physical bodies, our minds, or our emotions. It is, however, much finer, being the energy by which they function.

The second kind of samadhi, by way of comparison, occurs when, with our eyes open, we experience ourselves as that pure vitality. With our eyes open and in full contact with our senses, we see the whole universe as no different from this that we are. We understand that there is but one reality of which the whole universe is a demonstration. Then everywhere we look, we see the face of God.

At that point there is no difference between sitting in meditation or rising up from it. When, through grace, this awareness emerges and is reinforced through our practice, then the delight of transcendental consciousness becomes a constant feature in our awareness. Whether we are waking, dreaming, or in deep sleep, we experience this delight.

Then the whole world looks different. The *Mahartha-manjari* says that consciousness marks itself, like a sign, on the entire universe. This is its *mudra*. Mudra, which usually means a hand-gesture in meditation practice, here means the sign that consciousness imprints on all that it absorbs. It makes the presence of the absolute glisten even in a blade of grass. So wherever we go and whatever we encounter, we never cease to meet the divine.

Here there is a complete identification of "I" with the Self. We experience ourselves as the subject of every event, and everything we once experienced as an object becomes an expression of consciousness. There is no moment, whether in the beginning, middle, or end, which is not the Self, and we consider everything to be within us as we gaze upon it with our eyes wide open.

When we turn our attention inward, we perceive the external permeated with consciousness; when we turn towards the external, we see only the Self. Over and over again, we experience the awareness of the highest state, both inwardly and outwardly. Even these terms cease to be meaningful. This is why Abhinavagupta says, "It is Shiva himself . . . who is ever sparkling in my heart. It is his highest Shakti herself who is ever playing on the edge of my senses. The entire world gleams as the wondrous delight of pure I-consciousness. Indeed, I know not what the sound 'world' is supposed to refer to."

Universal Integration

The Tantric tradition is in no way life-denying. Rather, as Rudi used to say, it compels us to embrace all of life, with all its pleasure and pain, joy and sorrow. It tells us that only when we take life as a whole, integrating ourselves completely into that whole, do we have the potential for experiencing fulfillment and recognizing the highest potentiality that exists within us.

What we work toward, and what the practice *is*, in a very real way, is absorption. This is the idea of *vyapti*, or integration. We are absorbing into ourselves all the energies and all the apparent diversity of the universe in the process of universal integration, or *mahavyapti*. This is the real practice of recognizing that every experience is nothing but ourselves; nothing but the process of opening to and absorbing the energy of all experience as our own.

For each of us there are many different things to be internalized. Many things brew up together to make the liquor of our worldly lives. We internalize this and, in so doing, rise to the awareness of mahavyapti.

Then instead of compartmentalizing our individual lives and the universe into different segments, and thereby finding ourselves increasingly alienated from ourselves and everything else, the tradition encourages us to see ourselves as a whole, and to experience our desires and fears, our pleasure and pain, as aspects of that whole. Abhinavagupta says of this, "There is no true happiness, except that which is absorption into the emerging energy, the very sphere of serenity and great joy. Happiness is subject to limitations only to the extent that one ignores this fact."

When we talk about transcendence, we are talking about the transcendence of the personal and the individual. It is the recognition of the presence of the infinite and of our whole individual existence as an extension of that power. We also mean going beyond duality to integration. When we integrate ourselves with another person, what emerges? The experience of joy. How much more powerful, then, is the joy of our integration into Life Itself.

One of the important insights of the practitioners of Trika Yoga has been that the experiences in our lives are not a means to some gratification in a temporal sense, but rather a means of making an offering to the deities of the senses, and thereby pleasing them. That is, instead of gratifying the senses and keeping our attention focused externally, the point is to experience a deeper part of ourselves, to examine the place from which the feeling of pleasure emerges, and to come to a deeper understanding of the source of pleasure itself. It is to *this* that we are devoted. Through this devotion we are admitted into the inner sanctum of the Self.

There is a certain philosophy of enjoyment here. The insight of these people was that we want to pay attention to the joy inherent in all aesthetic experiences. Delving deeply into them, we see in all experience that subtle vibrancy and recognize it as nothing but our own consciousness. We experience the plentitude of our own being, and no longer think either, "I have it," or "I don't have it." Why would we, when everything is fullness?

Rather than pursuing pleasure through external modes of behavior we come to understand that, as beautiful as it may be to look for pleasure outside of ourselves, how much more extraordinary and beautiful is this inner life. The things that many people worship and pursue — money, drinking, sex, and all the sources of temporary pleasures — cannot hold a candle to the immense joy that exists within us. Thus these things are not to be denied; rather, handled properly and carefully, they are to be seen as vehicles toward the experience of something deeper and higher within us.

There is no question of sin, because everything has its place within the universal integration of mahavyapti. Depending on the awareness from which we pursue it, whatever we engage in can be an act of adoration. This is what determines the outcome. Just as money goes to money, anger to anger, hurt to more hurt, and violence to more violence, so love goes to love.

Even now we experience this depth all the time every day. Yet because it is a subtle event and we are not usually paying attention, we miss it. Perhaps, for example, we smell a flower or see something beautiful. In so doing, we may catch a glimpse of something precious, but our attention almost immediately goes off to the next thing. This happens to all of us.

Occasionally, however, something occurs that touches us profoundly. If, in those moments, we take our attention inside and release everything, we enter into the deeper experience of the simple joy within ourselves. This is the vehicle to the experience of divine joy. When we can do this, our senses are not obstacles at all.

The *Maharthamanjari* says there are five energies that are related to the world and the senses. These energies are represented as goddesses who stand at the gates of the inner sanctum at various points in the temple, and this is what is meant by the deities of the senses. It is a way of saying that we have to pass through these energies which, at one level, we experience as resistance and the source of our entanglement in desires and needs. This means that the senses do not deny us access to the Self, as some other schools of thought would claim. Here they are understood to be vehicles by which we can attain the experience of total well-being. We switch their polarity through our practice of meditation, that is, through internalizing our attention and stabilizing it there. In so doing, we reverse our focus.

Intense experiences of any kind, and all the sensations coming to us through every sense organ, can be significant points of reference for the intense energy at their core and at the very core of our existence. Abhinavagupta talks about this as the process of recognizing the source of any strong experience. The point is that all our intense experiences, underneath their direct content, are nothing but the energy of the divine.

What we are trying to do here is not to attain something foreign to us but to understand our own essence. Since each of us has the infinite creative energy of Life as our own essence, we can, with great confidence, engage in this discovery process. The senses are simply the mediators, or filters, of our creative energy. Through them this energy is articulated in various ways.

In *The Bhagavad Gita*, Krishna tells Arjuna to recognize that all existence, be it flowering and beautiful or wrathful and horrific, has its origin in the splendor of the divine. Thus there is no sensory experience that is not divine by its own nature. This is because the power of sensation is also the divine creative energy. The things we may think of as pleasurable, and therefore potentially sinful, also have the possibility of becoming vehicles through which we can experience and become established in the higher state.

In Trika Yoga there is no attempt to deny the senses or in any way withdraw from the objects of the senses, namely, the world. Here we embrace it all, participating in and recognizing our true relationship to it. In so doing we transcend both the objects of the senses and the senses themselves.

The *Maharthamanjari* says:

"When the yogin has understood that consciousness contains everything in itself, any activity, by the fact that it arises from this consciousness, becomes a rite of devotion. Under these conditions, why should one go to venerate Shiva in a temple? One's own body is a tabernacle and our own energies are divinities to be adored."

The question raised here is this: If all experience discloses the divine, then why go to a temple? We understand the reality of this notion if we practice daily. Slowly we realize not only that all our offerings are actually offerings of the Self, but that the receiver of the offerings is also the Self. Moreover, that which connects the two is the Self as well.

The finest level of our experience has an aesthetic substance to it. This is why many of the texts use one image after another to express the idea that every image we can possibly see is nothing more than a manifestation of the highest reality. When we become aware of this, how can we look at the rays of the sun without thinking "This is like that highest reality." When I sit down by the ocean and watch the waves moving across the water, I have the sense that the ocean is teaching me.

The same thing happens when we look at the birds, the trees, or the flowers that bloom. I see it even in watching the people with whom I share my life as they move around in the house. There are so many poignant moments that strike me, and their poignancy is nothing other than that highest state, which has merged into the experience of whatever we are observing.

All experience speaks to us with the voice of God. It says, "Look deeper. Look again." It encourages us to be aware of *seeing* when we look at things. It teaches us that there are levels of seeing, hearing, tasting, and touching. What we would call "the seasoning of the heart" is initiated through the experience of an aesthetic pleasure, in which we experience the beauty in every sensory experience and the well-being within that, understanding that such well-being is actually one. The essential injunction is to be aware.

When we enter into this awareness, we feel the delight and joy of the Self. We cannot help but transmit that sense of well-being to all those who come in contact with us. Think, after all, of what it is like for others to be around you when you feel completely happy. It is contagious. If that happiness were the delight taken from complete absorption into the Self, how could it not infuse the lives of others with delight?

Inadvertently, just by virtue of being, a person like this disseminates knowledge of the Self to those who encounter him or her. Every word becomes a mantra, every gesture a mudra. When "I" and the Self are one, this cannot be otherwise.

The Shaivite tradition does not conceive of the divine as creator of a universe distinct from itself through the power of the word but rather as an artist who cannot contain this sense of profound joy, and who must pour it forth as the universe in an infinite song or picture or poem. This is the manifestation of the world and the reality of the Self.

There is one more phase to this. Anavopaya, shaktopaya, and shambhavopaya are points along the same spectrum. Through our upward circulation of the energy, our awareness becomes refined to the extent that we have the capacity to surrender ourselves and allow that total, inner transformation. But when the ego's sense of separateness fully dissolves into the sense of one, there is real union, free of all desire and delusion, and of every residual sense of differentiation. This is called *anupaya*, or pure awareness, and it coincides with turyatita.

In one sense there is nothing to say about it because it refers to an awareness that has nothing to do with what we usually refer to with language. In this state our awareness of our awareness fuses in such a way that there is no longer any discernable object of awareness. All is Self, and there is only subject — no object. In other words, in anupaya, conscious-ness is extinguished as an object to itself. Then there is only pure awareness. There is also no fundamental distinction between pure consciousness and its expression. Then since there is only subject, and since awareness is infinite, there is not exactly any feedback.

When we try to focus and become aware of our own awareness, we find that we cannot do this and think at the same time. Certainly, in that state of ultimate awareness, which is referred to as *nirvikalpa samadhi*, or "samadhi without thought constructs," there are not two things, but only one. From the perspective of that state, we understand why things are referred to as an illusion all the way up to the highest state. At that point all of it disappears: body, senses, and awareness. All are seen as expressions of one thing.

Often, especially in the beginning, we think of ourselves as being on a spiritual path. When we meditate, we talk about "looking inside" to "open this" or "feel that." At that stage we think in terms of such objectives. This is true regardless of the specific practice. If it is Transcendental Meditation, one is hoping to realize a higher level of consciousness. If Buddhism, then perhaps one is searching to know what nirvana is. If Vedanta, one wants to know what is sometimes referred to as witness consciousness.

Kashmir Shaivism says, however, that Shiva may not be apprehended or known and that the witness is also not known. Having attained the highest state, we find there is nei-ther an object nor the absence of an object. This is a subtle point, but the gist of it is that the highest awareness is subtle and has no object. Rather our experience is one of the com-plete and infinite nature of our individual consciousness.

There is no object of awareness in that state. There is not even the reverberation of our own consciousness. We simply experience everything as ourselves, without classification or distinction. This has nothing to do with seeking or knowing, but only pure being. We find total well-being in stillness, and the stillness at the heart of a sense of total well-being. In this completely nondual event there is not even a different state of consciousness. There is no different feeling, no separate thought, nor anything distinct from ourselves by which we are to be uplifted.

This is the expression of the highest and finest possible state there is. It is also a state that is accessible to every human being because, in fact, we are nothing other than this. The person who lives in this awareness is said to be liberated in life or like God, because all forms of phenomena are sustained in that environment and no form is denied. More, even, than awareness of our awareness, this is pure awareness itself.

~~~~~~

Building a Spiritual Life

Eating, drinking, walking, standing — do not elevate the soul. Do your own work, do not desire to eat what others have cooked. With faith, do what you have to do.

— NITYANANDA

Generally speaking, people who are in pursuit of growing are exposed to a lot of talk about "the spiritual journey" or "the search." Often we hear about going beyond one thing or another, or reaching something else. In one sense this language is functional; in another it gives us the false sense that there is somewhere to go other than where we are. Not only that, but it suggests that upon arriving in that place we will be different from who we are now, and that life will be something other than what we now know it to be. All our warts will be removed without pain or strain. We will lose any amount of weight we want and, along the way, will develop innumerable talents and charms, even as we turn into a whole different ball of wax. All of this is quite incredible — and also a complete misunderstanding.

In a way it is problematic to talk about growth at all. The fact of the matter is that we are mining a treasure that is already there, discovering something in its fullness that is always present. Does the ocean "grow?" Likewise, the problem with the idea of phases of practice is that we are apt to think in terms of achievement. Then we may get cocky and start to slough off the things we have mastered. This only means we have not mastered anything, and we get sucked right back down.

We have to understand that the minute we get stuck in our minds and start trying to crack one phase or another, the possibility that we will once again embrace the whole dualistic aspect of creation springs right back into the foreground. Just as the possibility for extraordinary awareness is always present, so is the tendency toward crystallization. We always confront the possibility of denying the whole for the sake of some aspect of its creative potential — a possibility which, in every case, sets us up to get whacked.

It doesn't matter how slick and fancy we are, or how sophisticated, informed, developed, and evolved. We are still going to get our noses broken. So from our perspective there is always only one thing articulating itself as a state of total well-being. For the sake of discussion, it is all right to make distinctions. In reality, however, when we are dealing with infinity, we have nothing but infinity. All this discussion is really a matter of intellectual manipulation done for our own enjoyment. When we know this, then such phases have no real hold on us.

At the same time, if we are aware that these phases will characterize various moments of our experience, then as we go from one atmosphere to another, we don't get lost and think, "Oh my God, I don't know what's going on here," or "This is a big change, and I'm suffering and dying."

Nor is it that big a deal to talk about phases. We can say that various levels of awareness have always operated in our lives as we have passed from one age to another. Finally, however, we recognize that underlying all these levels, and present at every single stage, was the fundamental creator of Life Itself, manifesting its own grace, talent, and will in the form of our individuated lives. Then we see that all distinct lives are nothing but an expression of one Life. We understand that there are no levels to this journey but only phases in the preparation of a painter's canvas or a sculptor's stone. All are parts of one creative process.

This recognition cuts through the problem of bringing one experience into line with another. It frees us from the need to carry the baggage of our past with us as we work to discover the creative content of our future. Past and future, we discover, are nothing but the same creative power pulsating with vitality and articulating its content in multiple ways.

In any discussion of the phases of practice, there are two schools of thought. The *Shiva Sutras* presents both of them simply and beautifully. First of all, by its division into sections pertaining to the different phases of practice, the very structure of the text pays lip service to the existence of such levels.

At the same time, within each of these sections are at least one or two sutras that fold back on the preceding level. In this way even the most sophisticated phase of awareness is immediately integrated back into the most contracted. There is an unbroken progression which is internally consistent with itself at every point. The underlying issue is whether there is succession or not. Do we grow in stages, or does realization happen in a flash? One approach says that it takes place in an instant. The other talks about a progression in our search for truth.

Both are right. At each and every moment, the highest awareness of one without other is always present. But, because of its own vitality, it also generates the appearance of levels. This is what makes our awakening both gradual and immediate. Each of the strategies merges into the other. They are all interconnected. Rudi described their relationship as a set of planes. He said that there were two horizontal planes: one material, the other transcendent. He suggested that there was a vertical plane that functioned as the intermediary between these two. Drawing on the language of his training in engineering, he was describing the relationship between anavopaya and shambhavopaya as the two horizontal planes, integrated through shaktopaya as the vertical plane. Each phase is a part of a continuum, a point in the creative display that manifests from within the highest self-awareness.

Through the Eyes of God

The notion of levels represents our experience of the different tones, shades, moods, and subtle vibrations in the various manifestations of energy within and around us. We appreciate and respect this by viewing all experience through the eyes of God. If we can do this, we will never lose our sense of what is important.

You might say that this sounds a bit difficult, but in fact it is not. Nothing I tell you is particularly difficult. To view everything with the eyes of God is simply to quiet our minds and to center our awareness in that vital power that is our inner spirit and the essence of our existence. We allow the logic of love to rise up in our hearts, permeate our minds, and shine out through our eyes. Because we cultivate the expansion of this inner light within us, it shines forth. We discover that the eyes of God are really our own, and that what sees within us is nothing but the divine itself shining.

In a way, building a spiritual life like this is something like raising a building. Clearing the site is analogous to straightening out our physical lives and making them simple. The basics of our practice — our sitting, breathing, and concentration — are the tools we use to dig out the masses of tension and misunderstanding on which our lives are usually constructed. Then there is a foundation to be poured, which must be well laid. Level by level, floor by floor, we raise our lives as a whole. We go from one vantage point to another within the same structure.

The difference in building a house is that once we do one thing, it is finished. Then we go on to the next thing, and the next. Building a spiritual life is just the opposite. We learn to deal with one thing, then two, then three. Gradually we learn to manage more and more. It is the same as the creative process of Life Itself.

Furthermore, we are not building something new. In this process we call growing, what we are reaching for is not something different from where we are now. Rather it is a more complete participation in the authentic reality that is always present. This reality evaporates our past and reveals the future to be an illusion. It is an understanding that not only allows, but also respects, the existence of all diversity. Nor is it a reductionist approach: We are not reducing everything to some small notion of consciousness. Instead, we are admiring the way in which this simple, dynamic stillness takes on an amazing diversity of form while remaining one thing.

From the grossest level of manifestation to the simplest pure experience of the Self there is a complete unity that is unbroken. It is from our own state of complete surrender and absolute nonattachment (vira vairagya) that we receive and unfold our own infinite creative Self in every level of manifestation. In our capacity as spiritual people we should have an ever-increasing ability to surrender our individuality and to observe our own consciousness functioning under our own actions.

To do so we have to get out of the way, so that our lives become a ritual in which we are participating not for our own gratification or enrichment but, even more subtly, as a recognition of our full participation in our total environment. This is our surrender. It is what teaches us how to look through the eyes of God.

Living in a state of surrender, we do things for love only. This is the basis of our integrity. It is what removes the blocks, difficulties, and struggles from the life of the sincere person. Whatever the level of our capacity, the ability we may bring to bear, or the degree of intensity we sustain in our practice, this integrity gives us the support, the strength, and the time it takes to do our work in this lifetime.

This makes us responsible for the form of our own lives. We are required to face things straight away, changing what we can and accepting what we must. This, however, in no way represents a problem. It is simply part of the process of allowing the finest level of creative energy to come into being through our surrender, and to enter into the field of our everyday, differentiated existence.

To have insight into the highest level of reality and to have contact with it on a daily basis in no way alters the reality of our physical existence. In this context, however, we begin to recognize ourselves as multidimensional events. This multidimensionality is part of a whole dynamic unity in which there is no real separation. Therefore, there is a reciprocal, balanced relationship between the highest level of self-awareness and the densest level of our physical existence.

Our spiritual evolution can only take place in a mental environment that is relatively stable and in which the interest in knowledge is stronger than the attachment to pleasure or the aversion to pain. A person who really knows God wants nothing else — indeed, wants nothing at all. The applause and recognition of human beings at that point is ridiculous because people often say anything to get what they want. That is not a cynical statement, but simply an observation about the kind of creatures we are.

Our identification with the universality of our own nature gives us a different perspective on the nature of our entire ordinary reality. As an experience it has a real, tangible effect. It is an energy event that literally changes the pattern, frequency, and chemistry of our being. For one thing, the observation of the subtle connectedness snaps our head around. We emerge simpler people, more reserved in our willingness to judge, less inclined to seek security in some temporary condition. For another, it gives rise to a deep sense of conviction.

Every day, we bring spiritual awareness into ourselves and demonstrate this awareness in our lives. When we can do this, we also demonstrate an extraordinary state of surrender in which we are able to absorb the feedback that is ever present in our environment. We digest that, change in the appropriate way, and improve our performance as a whole. This articulation of our skills in the process of losing ourselves is a heroic endeavor. This is what brings us to an awareness of every subtle dimension of existence from its source.

Doing Our Own Work

Everything I have been saying about our practice — about releasing tensions and allowing our creative energy to flow — can only happen if we do the work. This has nothing to do with the forms our lives take. Nor is there ever any real issue of what someone else did, is doing, or is going to do, but only of what *we* are going to do. This is the one issue of any importance. It is our individual work that matters.

What other people do to affect our lives is irrelevant. What this one has done to us or that one has failed to do for us has nothing to do with anything. The real issue is this: What will *we* do now? We have to know and do from the deepest part of ourselves, and start to articulate that power in the deepest extension possible. We then articulate it in the whole field of our lives.

The onus continually falls back on our ability to release tensions and allow the creative energy in every situation to flow. It depends on our ability to use our own experience of this flow to guide us to a state of stillness, and then to participate in the situation from that perspective. It is up to us to sustain our awareness of this stillness even as we move through our everyday lives, functioning from it both graciously and gracefully as much as possible. We try to be strong and clear in every case. In this way we develop from the depth of ourselves an experience of Life that is truly miraculous and magical. Moreover, we have the capacity to extend that magic and miracle into the lives of the people around us.

This is real work. Rudi understood this well. He said that growth *means* hard work. The vision he once had of himself as a water buffalo walking endlessly around an enormous grindstone was an expression of the enormity of the work he knew he would have to do in his lifetime. He said that the need to relax from this work was only for those who wanted childish rewards.

We have to cultivate the strength, comfort, and stability within ourselves to do this work at all times. Otherwise our capacity to bring about change and deal with discomfort not only in ourselves, but in others, will be extremely limited. If we are not fundamentally centered and established in our own inner work, all the changes around us will overset us. First we become agitated, then we react. By that time we can forget it, because the chaos has passed over into our own hands. Next we are the ones generating all the tension until, finally, the system surrounding us kicks us back into line.

Few of us are willing to face the enormity of the task, and none of us can complete it until we have learned to connect every day to the ultimate resource inside us. If we allow that resource to permeate our existence as a flow of creative energy, we enter into a state where that energy can flow, purifying our hearts and minds, our relationships and actions. Then instead of a destructive event we have one that is a kind of rebirth. Such an experience, after a few times, instills in us a profound sense of confidence.

This is in no way the same thing as arrogance. We also recognize that many highly improbable things can occur, so our experience does not allow us to become arrogant. We have seen the improbable happen too many times. We can, however, be steady, quiet, and at peace. We can recognize an elegance that manifests as a continuous sense of rebirth. At the same time we experience an extension in our range of self-expression that lies within the deepest heart of a human being. When this is so, it does not matter what difficulty arises. Each such moment is also the occasion for quiet, stability, and steadiness.

None of this means that tensions ever go away. There is an endless supply that will continue to be present throughout our lives. What does happen, however, is that these tensions no longer provoke any kind of discharge from us, nor do they inhibit our field of function. This is important, because in many people's minds, discharge and release are synonymous. So we take one day at a time and make the effort to avoid getting caught up in all the things that represent opportunities for tension, doubt, and entanglement.

Given how quickly agitation can flare up, we become observant of ourselves, and simple and clear about our work, so that we become better able to transcend these tensions on a daily basis. Only by dealing successfully with our own nonsense over and over again to the point where it takes not two hundred years but just four seconds will we ever develop the capacity to help anyone else resolve their confusions.

It is the job of a spiritual person to draw tensions from others. This is, finally, the ultimate act of surrender. When it is said that Jesus died for people's sins, what does this really mean? All other issues aside, sins are really just tensions and the withholding of love. It was Jesus' willingness to take on the tensions of others and to consume them within himself that was his service, his sacrifice, and his surrender.

As people committed to growing, we cannot reject other people's tensions, or even react to them, except with love and respect. The degree to which we are settled, calm within ourselves, and simply aware is the degree to which we will be able to facilitate this creative process whenever and wherever we find ourselves.

It is within our power, in every case, to change the nature of any dynamic event. We can do so either in a physical sense by making some concrete effort, or in a spiritual sense by changing the level on which we relate to it. This we do for long enough that the new vibration establishes itself in our understanding of the event and in our behavior.

As we advance in our practice, every day we make the effort not to do the easy thing — not to succumb to the ignorance — but to do the great and intelligent thing. We make the effort to go into our hearts and open ourselves completely to our lives, to our Self, and to all the forms in which this manifests: to all the people, places, and events we attract to ourselves. These are all occasions for our inner work so, ultimately, it doesn't matter what they are.

What does matter is the depth of the openness we bring to each moment and the work we do to transform every experience into one that makes us feel closer to our Self, more in contact with our own lives, and more in touch with the presence of God. It is not that we reduce God to some event like ourselves, but that we rise above our individuality to attain the knowledge and understanding of the biggest picture that exists and to live in that big picture.

Living continuously in that big picture is what is sometimes called enlightenment. It doesn't mean that the world is destroyed but that we permanently and completely rise above it. It doesn't mean that pain and tensions stop; it does mean that they don't touch us in the same way because we no longer live immersed in that level. Even if we happen to pass through them accidentally, we have enough sense not to stay very long.

This understanding comes about from practice and patience. When we are willing to do the work within the simplicity of the state to which we aspire, we discover a subtlety and sophistication that are, in themselves, both dazzling and compelling. They inspire us to continue in our quest to understand this creative energy, the matrix of vitality from which all creative energy and all manifestation have emerged. Thus it all comes back to spanda.

Then there only remains the clarity, joy, and extraordinary sense of peace and fulfillment that characterizes the experience of authentic living. We recognize that every shift in our awareness teaches us about surrender, just as every surrender teaches about another shift. We find that we are practicing for no reason, but simply as a way of life. Our practice now shapes what we are. We do it not as a way to get anything, but as a way of being. It becomes what we do for its own sake.

We can never be fully prepared for what this will require of us, because we don't know in advance what we are getting into. It is like being a parent: How on earth can anyone be fully prepared beforehand to be a mother or a father? On the most basic level, we do not even know each day if we will live or die. This may seem overly dramatic — after all, we probably have some idea of what we will be doing later today, and next week — but just because we are familiar with the road doesn't mean the risks are not there. Traveling it in a state of complete surrender is what enables us to appreciate the potential within each moment.

I suspect that what often turns people away from pursuing a spiritual life in the first place is our system's innate resistance to engaging in the extraordinary depth and degree of work, change, and reorganization that take place in our field of awareness. We anticipate that life as we know it will come to an end — and it will. Yet this is no real reason for not doing the work.

I cannot say that there may not be something beyond the range of consciousness. Maybe there is. But as far as we are concerned (and this appears to have been the experience of the great spiritual masters), there is nothing greater than that. As far as these people have been able to travel, they have never found anything other or greater than this.

This suggests that as human beings we will never find anything other than consciousness. We may find finer and finer realms of conscious activity, but it has been my experience that it is impossible to go beyond consciousness itself. So to arrive at the point where we recognize the infinite nature of our individual consciousness does not represent an end to anything. Rather it represents the beginning of what is perhaps the most extraordinary and intense endeavor upon which any human being can embark. Thus it is somewhat wrong to think that we arrive at the awareness of infinity as an end point to our work. It is not like that.

My ultimate conclusion, in this regard, is that there is some force — although I haven't the words to describe it to you — something within us that moves us when we are able to get out of the way and allow it to do so. I don't think any human being has the sense, otherwise, to pull him- or herself up out of the soup in which most of us swim around. We would not think to move toward something finer and deeper on our own. Indeed, this may be the last choice that we grab hold of.

Yet there is some force that stirs within us, independent of our wills. For that matter, it continues to stir, no matter how many times and how many different ways we bend, twist, and shred it. It continues to compel us to want to know, to grow, and to try to understand.

This is an extraordinary thing, because it is not really *us* doing it. I know that the passion I have for living and for growing is not something that I chose. Rather it is simply there, and I am discovering the depth and breadth of it on a daily basis. It is this which expresses itself in our commitment to growing and which brings about within us the capacity to cut through confusion. From this there emerges the clarity that allows us to participate in the logic of love, the logic by which we are able to extend ourselves beyond our boundaries every day to participate in the experience of universal integration.

Without that logic of love, we will tremble in fear before our vision of the infinite. We will experience ourselves only as separate from that, and see in the vision of the infinite only our own demise. The logic of the world will cause us to run from the experience of integration because we will have the illusion that there is something we will lose and something we will suffer.

Yet the logic of love is, in a way, no logic at all. It is, instead, an experience of such fullness that we look into the infinite and see ourselves. We feel into the infinite and find such joy that we can barely hold ourselves together. In this experience we, like the sufi in Rumi's poem, beg each moment to give our lives away. We discover that all real spiritual exercises, irrespective of their level of subtlety, only make sense in the context of the experience of surrender. That is, they only begin to have some kind of real meaning and depth of sophistication when that surrender is present. Otherwise they are only so many mechanical techniques.

Some of that does have an effect. Breathing exercises, for example, can intensify the pulsation of the cerebrospinal fluid and have a beneficial effect on a number of levels. But to talk about refining our practice, even if I were to give you some advanced techniques, makes no sense when surrender is not present. Moreover, when surrender is present, we do not need techniques or explanations. All these things simply become absorbed into our blood.

If you can take this one point to heart and make it the guiding principle of your life, you then have the means to attain everything. Without it you can possess every technique and initiation and have read everything in the world, and you still will have nothing of lasting value.

Instead, it is our patience and perseverance as we surrender the individual into the infinite that releases every tension, overcomes every obstacle and difficulty, severs every knot, and brings us to perfection. This is a matter of what Rudi called the equation for spiritual growth: Real growth is a function of depth, over time. The discussion, finally, closes upon the issue of our resolve to grow. In our efforts as human beings and our participation in every level of life, we must continuously rediscover that resolve, which we could just as well call balance, or commitment. All of these are the same thing.

It is only in that ultimate state of surrender that we experience love, for what is love, anyway, but ultimate self-surrender? This self-surrender brings a profound and total experience of renewal. The power of this is not something that can be understood or analyzed, and there is no message within it. It gives no support to any particular form or direction in our lives, because love is so vast as to be beyond any real discussion or description. Still, we have spiritual practices and spiritual teachers to nourish and support us until we come to that point where we simply release everything.

It is in that complete release that universal love reveals itself to our minds, and through our bodies, into the world. There are many ways to pursue the experience of this love, even though, in a way, it is not pursuable at all. Nevertheless it always remains our endeavor.

In my opinion, it is the only endeavor that will always add value to our lives. Any undertaking without it only brings about some measure of depreciation. This doesn't mean that we should never relax and have fun. In fact, an important part of our work is to make everything fun, no matter how difficult it is. In every situation we want to find the joy and experience it. The point is not to do so at the expense of our attention.

During the time we have in this world, we make it the point of our lives to experience and attempt to understand the creative power within us. We must do so if our lives are ever to have any lasting value at all. I do not think there can be anything more important for a human being than the pursuit of this love and joy. Therefore, in whatever way you choose to look for it in the course of your own life, I sincerely wish you well.

Glossary

The following is a glossary of names and terms used in Parts One and Two of *Dynamic Stillness*. All italicized words are defined.★

a

Abhinavagupta The most famous and probably the greatest sage-philosopher of Kashmir Shaivism. He lived in the second half of the 10th century and the first quarter of the 11th century C.E. He was the fourth in succession from *Somananda* in a line of spiritual discipleship.

Abhinavagupta is widely recognized as the central theoretician of Indian aesthetics. His various writings on drama, dance, poetry, and music have had a lasting influence on the appreciation of these disciplines. He was also a profound mystic and mastered the doctrines of the orthodox schools of Indian philosophy in the process of arriving at his own comprehensive philosophical synthesis. In this area his most famous work is the *Tantraloka*.

Advaita Vedanta *Advaita* means "not two," and *Vedanta* means "end of the Veda." Vedanta was originally the name given to the Vedic philosophy of the *Upanishads*, the last group of Vedic writings, which take Vedic philosophical speculation to its highest phase. Later the name became associated with

★Glossary based on *Glossary of Terms Commonly Used in Kashmir Shaivism*, compiled by Joan Ames (Cambridge: Nityananda Institute, 1990).

the *Advaita Vedanta* of the teachers Gaudapada and Sham-
karacharya (about the 8th century C.E.).

This philosophy stresses the unity of the Self (*Atman*)
and the Absolute (*Brahman*). It teaches that consciousness,
or *Brahman*, is the only reality and that everything else is
manifested by false impressions based on beginningless
ignorance (*avidya*).

agama Lit., "tradition." A revealed text or traditional knowledge. A traditional doctrine or sacred work, or a collection
of such doctrines. Held to be divinely inspired, authored by
the divine, and handed down from generation to generation. Also a *Tantra*, or work related to the teachings of *Shiva*
and *Shakti*.

The *agamas*, or agamic texts, are perhaps the most important sources for all the Shaiva traditions. As revelations
handed down from teacher to pupil, these scriptures began
to appear perhaps as early as the 4th century C.E., and
almost certainly by the 7th or 8th century C.E. The material
in these texts is aimed at transmitting the means of awakening to the highest awareness rather than setting forth meta-
physical speculation. They lay out the doctrines and
practices of the system. At the same time, they also contain
information on the history of Indian spirituality and philosophy, as well as on the history of Indian art. Among the
agamas of Kashmir Shaivism is the *Vijnanabhairava*.

aham I, or I-ness. Consciousness of the true Self. The beholding subject. The supreme "I" and the primordial *mantra*.

ahamkar Ego; the I-making principle. The part of the mind
particularly associated with the mantra of stupidity, "What's
going to happen to me?"

ajapa-japa See *hamsa*.

akasha Lit., "sky." Space, heart space. A symbol of pure consciousness, also translated as the sky, or infinite; the subtlest
of the five elements into which all elements ultimately
resolve; ether.

ananda Total well-being; often rendered as "bliss." The essential principle of joy unaffected by worldly objects. The

nature of *Shakti*. Along with *sat* ("being"), and *chit* ("consciousness"), these qualities describe the Absolute.

anavopaya or **anava upaya** One of the four *upayas*, or strategies in the process of Self-realization, described in the *Shiva Sutras*. The strategy of individual effort, characterized by dualistic thinking (*abheda* or *apara*).

animation, four states of 1) *jagrat*, waking; 2) *svapna*, dreaming; 3) *sushupti*, the deep sleep state, or dreamless sleep; 4) *turya*, self-revelation. *Turyatita*, the transcendent state, is sometimes considered the fifth state of animation.

anupaya or **ananda yoga** The highest *yoga*. This is not usually considered to be a separate *upaya*, but is described as *shambhavopaya* in its highest and most mature phase. Spontaneous realization of the *Self* without any special effort.

anusamdhana Lit., "investigation"; tracking a matter to its source. In *yoga*, the repeated intensive awareness of the source of all experience, or essential reality. Particularly pertinent in the discussion of going beyond sensory perceptions and psychological states, for example.

apara Lower or lowest; immanent. When it lies dormant in three and a half folds around the lowest *chakra*, the *kundalini shakti* is known as *apara*, simply immanent in life, not yet active. Bringing about a sense of difference.

Arjuna One of the five Pandava brothers and an important figure in the Indian epic *The Mahabharata*. He is well known as *Krishna's* beloved disciple and friend from *The Bhagavad Gita*, a popular excerpt from the epic.

asana Posture, in *hatha yoga*; seat. *Yoga* aims at focus and one-pointedness. *Hatha yoga* is included in this step. The exoteric meaning refers to a particular posture of the body; the esoteric meaning, to being established in the *Self*.

Atman The *Self*; spirit; eternal principle present in the heart of every living being.

avidya Ignorance; beginningless ignorance.

b

Bhagavad Gita *Bhagavan* means "Lord," and *Gita* means "song." "The Song of the Lord." A portion of *The Mahabharata* and one of the great works of spiritual literature in which *Krishna*, the incarnation of Lord *Vishnu*, explains the path of liberation to his chosen devotee, *Arjuna*, on the battlefield of the war described in the epic poem.

Bhagavan Godhead; one who is full of light; Lord.

bhakti Ardent devotion and love of God.

Bhairava Undifferentiated *Shiva*. The highest reality, or *para*. Bhairava is the form of *Shiva* most often encountered in the non-dual Kashmir Shaivite texts. Representations of this aspect of God show a form of dread and terror. A sinister, fanged face often surmounted by writhing serpents conveys the fury of the god of uncertainty, destruction, and death. At the same time, upon closer examination, the same face is discovered to be smiling, as this is also the god of regeneration and renewal. The multiple aspects represented in the same figure suggest that it is our perspective that determines which aspect predominates in our own awareness.

Bhairava mudra A state in which the attention is established within, even as one gazes upon the world with open eyes, fully in contact with one's senses.

bheda Difference, diversity. Refers to the awareness characteristic of *anavopaya*.

bhedabheda Unity in diversity. Refers to the awareness of *shaktopaya*.

bija A phonic seed. The active light of the highest *Shakti*, which is the root cause of the universe; vowel; the mystical letter forming the essential part of the sacred word (mantra); the first syllable of a sacred word.

bija mantra Mantras formed from syllables that have no conventional meaning, *i.e.*, meaningless syllables. The heart mantra, *sauh*, is an example. Each of the smallest units of speech (phonemes) in a *bija mantra* can be given a symbolic meaning. This may then be used as a code for the mantra in texts where the author does not want to spell out the actual sacred word.

bindu A drop, dot. In the pulsation of the highest reality there are parameters known as bindus, or stillpoints. Here the universe-to-be lies in its full potentiality. It is the fullness of *Shiva* gathered up in an undifferentiated point, on the verge of manifesting. A point without dimension, a symbol of *Shiva* undifferentiated.

Brahma The god of creation. Brahma is the creator, Vishnu the preserver or sustainer, and *Shiva* the dissolver or destroyer. Together these three make up the different aspects of the divine. Although they are sometimes referred to as the Hindu trinity, they are all aspects of one highest reality.

Brahman The Vedantic term for the absolute reality, the power of the sacrifice; the divine ground of existence. Becomes a more comprehensive term — the ultimate, absolute reality of the universe, the impersonal godhead; the highest reality. In *Advaita Vedanta* this is the pure foundational consciousness without activity; unlimited knowledge devoid of activity. In Shaiva philosophy, it is the pure foundational consciousness full of omniscience and omnipotence, the One.

buddhi The understanding capacity; the intellect; the ascertaining intelligence; the steady, or higher, mind; a faculty higher than manas; the capacity or faculty of subtle discrimination and ascertainment; spiritual discernment; decision and will; intelligent will; the superpersonal mind; the intuitive aspect of consciousness by which the essential *Self* awakens to truth; wisdom.

c

chakra Lit., "wheel"; the vibratory centers of conscious energy in the subtle body through which the life energy (*kundalini*) moves. Most scriptures cite seven: 1) base of the spine, 2) sexual organs, 3) navel, 4) heart, 5) throat, 6) forehead, and

7) the crown of the head. The chakras are associated with three channels: the central *sushumna*, flanked on the left and right by the *ida* and *pingala nadis*. These nerves and centers are not biological. When the *kundalini* is awakened, it travels up the *sushumna*, passing through the *chakras*. Consciousness widens as each higher *chakra* is crossed, until the highest state is realized when the *kundalini* energy merges with its source, the energy of Life Itself, in the *chakra* at the crown of the head.

chetana Consciousness; consciousness intermediate between the highest level and the ordinary empirical consciousness; the *Self*; the soul; the conscious individual; pure Self-awareness.

Chetanananda *chetana* + *ananda*: The bliss, or total well-being, of pure Self-awareness.

chidakasha *chit*, absolute consciousness + *akasha*, subtle inner space; thus, "sky of consciousness." In the *sutras* of *Nityananda*, this is translated, alternately, as sky of the heart, heart-sky, and heart-space.

chit The Absolute; foundational consciousness. Along with being (*sat*), and bliss (*ananda*), these qualities describe the infinite. The unchanging principle of all change. One caveat: The problem with translating *chit* as "consciousness" is that consciousness implies a subject and an object; in other words, a knower and something that is known. *Chit*, however, is not relational. The changeless principle of all changing experience, it is pure awareness; an immediacy of feeling in which neither "I" nor "this" is distinguished.

chitta In the *Trika Yoga* system, the empirical mind of the individual in the broad sense of mental, or psychic apparatus. It consists of *buddhi*, the discriminative intelligence that gives name and meaning to the perceptions of *manas*; *ahamkar*, the I-consciousness of the individual that acts as a self-appropriating intelligence; and *manas*, the perceiving intelligence that, with the senses, builds up perceptions and images — the limited mind.

Chitta is the limitation of the universal consciousness manifesting as the individual mind. In general English usage, "mind" is often used as a synonym for both chitta as well as the more limited manas.

d

darshan Lit., "seeing." Intuitive vision. Revelation or intuitive experience of the truth brought about by the practice of yoga. The act of seeing the divinity within the *guru* or within a representation of the divine, as in a sculpture or painting. A system of philosophy. Going to see and be seen by the *guru* or the figure of the deity.

diksha The gift of spiritual knowledge; the initiation ceremony in which the *guru* imparts spiritual knowledge to the student and purifies the residual traces of his or her former deeds.

dualism The condition of being twofold, or not one. In contrast to *monism*, the view that the world consists of more than one thing, such as mind and matter. In some religious traditions, the idea that the world is ruled by antagonistic forces of good and evil. The concept that a human being has two basic natures, the physical and the spiritual.

dukkha Suffering; pain.

f

five activities of the divine Creation, preservation, dissolution, self-obscuration, and self-recognition.

g

granthi Lit., "knot." Psychic tangle; psychic complex. Three points of focus within the system of *chakras*.

guna/gunas Quality, property, attribute; the three primary constituents of the basic substance of manifest reality. Gunas are qualities which create the sense of individualization. Part of the system of tattvas, as one enters the discussion of manifestation.

guru A channel or medium of the grace-bestowing power of the divine. A perfected spiritual master who has realized identity with the highest reality, and who can impart this experience to a student.

h

hamsa Lit., "swan," "goose." Symbol of the *Self.* The breath mantra. The inhalation sounding inaudibly as "ha" and exhalation sounding inaudibly as "sah," along with the nasal sound "am" at the junction point. Together these form "ham-sah." This is known as nonrecited recitation (*ajapa-japa*), because every living being repeats it constantly and automatically without any conscious effort. When a person consciously practices this, it is known as the *hamsa mantra.* By conscious repetition, it is converted into *so'ham* ("I am That, *i.e., Shiva*).

hatha yoga A method of attaining awakening by employing the vital energy flowing through the *nadis*; in this *yoga*, great importance is given to physical strength and flexibility.

hrid/hridaya Heart, the mystic center. An important center, or *chakra.* The light of central consciousness, which is the underlying reality of all manifestation. When referring to *prana*, or breath, *hridaya* can also mean the center of the diaphragm.

i

iccha Divine will. Desire, impulsion.

iccha-shakti The power of will or being; one of the three fundamental forces or powers of the energy of Life Itself, the others being the power of knowledge (*jnana-shakti*) and the power of action (*kriya-shakti*). The inseparable innate will power of the highest reality intent on manifestation; that inward state of that highest reality, in which knowledge and action are unified. The predominant aspect of the divine.

ida One of the three primary *nadis*, or channels, for the energy flow in the subtle body. The *ida* begins on the left and with its counterpart, the *pingala*, crisscrosses over the central *sushumna*. All three intersect at the seven major *chakras*, and culminate in the *chakra* at the crown of the head.

j

japa Recitation, resonance related to inner utterance. A devotional exercise consisting in the repetition of a mantra or the name of a deity. The Christian equivalent might be the saying of the rosary.

jivanmukta One liberated while yet alive (*jivan*, while living + *mukti*, liberation). The liberated individual who while still living in the physical body is not conditioned by the limitation of his or her subtle and gross constitution, and who experiences the entire universe to be an expression of the *Self*, or *Shiva*.

jnana Knowledge; limited knowledge that is the source of bondage; spiritual wisdom; the *Shakti* of *Shiva*.

jnana-shakti The power of wisdom or knowing, one of the three fundamental powers of the energy of Life Itself along with *iccha-shakti* and *kriya-shakti*.

jnana yoga See *shaktopaya*.

k

Kabir A great poet-saint who lived his life as a weaver in Benares (1440-1518). His followers were both Hindus and Moslems.

kanchuka/kanchukas Sheaths, or cloaks. The five principles of subjective limitation, the five *kanchukas* are five powers of the Absolute in their contracted, individualized expression.

These are the limiting *tattvas* that cloak and cover pure consciousness, as part of the crystallizing of *Shiva* into the individualized self.

These are 1) the limitation of omnipotence into individual agency, 2) the limitation of omniscience into finite knowledge, 3) the limitation of infinite will into specific desires, 4) the limitation of infinity into spatial and causal relationships (these first four limit a person's field of knowing and doing), 5) the limitation of infinity into the experience of time (this limits a person's very being).

karikas Verses.

karma Act, action, performance, business; work, labor. Actions performed with some expectation or with the desire for some outcome. The element of attachment leads to the accumulation of residues — we could say tensions — that are said to keep a person bound to the cycle of death and rebirth. Also, the law of causation governing action and its effects; moral law. From the perspective of the highest reality there is no such thing, because there is no causality.

Kashmir Region of northern India where the nondualistic philosophy called Kashmir Shaivism, with its different branches, developed and flourished. One of these was the practice and philosophy of *Trika Yoga*.

krama mudra Mystical attitude equalizing inner and outer experience. The condition in which the mind, totally absorbed in the *Self*, moves alternately between the internal, the essential *Self*, and the external, the world which now also appears as *Shiva*, or the *Self*.

Krishna Lit., "the dark one"; the one who attracts irresistibly. The eighth incarnation of the god *Vishnu*, whose life story is described in *The Mahabharata*, and whose teachings to *Arjuna* are contained in *The Bhagavad Gita*. He is often worshipped in the form of a child. As a young man, he was adored by all the village cowherd girls, especially Radha. The romance between the two of them symbolizes the lover-beloved relationship that the devotee may have with the Lord.

kriya Activity, action. The power of activity.

Kshemaraja An eleventh century student of Abhinavagupta. Little is known about his life, although some scholars speculate that he was a cousin of Abhinavagupta. A prolific writer credited with commentaries on most of the major sources of the *Trika* system.

kundalini Lit., "coiled up." The creative power of *Shiva*, that aspect of *Shakti* that lies coiled in three and a half folds in the *chakra* at the base of the spine. The subtle power of animation moving upward through the spine experienced by yogins during the experience of the well-being of the *Self*. This *shakti* can be awakened by a *guru* through the process of *shaktipat*. The main aim of spiritual practice is to rouse this power in oneself and cause it to pass through the *chakras* in the *sushumna*. The energy moves successively through the *chakras* and finally dissolves in the crown *chakra*.

l

linga/lingam Lit., a "sign"; sometimes revered in the form of special stones tumbled by river currents into the form of a long egg. 1) As the symbol of *Shiva*, the *linga* is a symbol of infinite potentiality, and therefore of dynamic stillness. As an aniconic symbol of *Shiva's* formless form, it is worshiped in temples. 2) The subtle space containing the whole universe in the process of formation and dissolution. 3) An erect phallus, also a symbol of potency and dynamic stillness.

m

Mahabharata, The The greatest ancient Indian epic, composed from two to three thousand years ago in oral tradition, and eventually written down. Traditionally attributed to the sage Vyasa, it relates the conflict between the descendents of Pandu, the forces of light, and those of Dhritarashtra, the forces of darkness. Contains eighteen books, including *The Bhagavad Gita*, and has been the source of countless literary and artistic renderings over the centuries in Indian culture.

mahartha The greatest end; the highest value; profound meaning; the pure I-consciousness. *Mahartha* also refers to the Krama school which arose in Kashmir towards the end of the 7th and beginning of the 8th century C.E.

Maharthamanjari A philosophical poem and commentary by the 12th century sage Maheshvarananda, also known as Goraksha, who was a follower of the Shaivism of Kashmir. *Mahartha* means the "profound meaning" and *manjari* means "a spray of flowers." The title is thus translated as "The Flowering of Ultimate Truth."

manas The internal sense, the empirical mind; the limited mind; that aspect of the mental apparatus that coordinates the perceptions of the senses, bringing these images and perceptions back to the subtle body. It is then the function of *buddhi* to discriminate among the images and discern their meaning.

mantra The syllable *man* means "reflect," or "be aware." The syllable *tra* means "agent of," "means for," or "tool for." A mantra is then a means of mentation, a tool of thought, a means of reflection. A sacred word or formula to be chanted; formulated to awaken the spiritual energy by constant repetition. A *mantra* is normally given by a *guru* to the student according to his or her predisposition.

In *shaktopaya,* that sacred word or formula by which the nature of the supreme is reflected on as identical with the *Self.* It is called *mantra* because it induces reflection on the highest reality and because it provides protection from the cycle of rebirth. In *shaktopaya*, the mind (*chitta*) itself assumes the resonance of *mantra*.

matrika The unknown mother; the divine source, or origin; the power of letters and words that is the basis of all knowledge; the highest *shakti* that generates the world. The source of all the *mantras*. Likewise, the source of both all confusion and all understanding.

maya From *ma*, to measure. Lit., "that which measures"; 1) the power that measures or limits; 2) in the *Trika*, the cosmic process or limiting force of the infinite that is responsible for the sense of duality. One of the *tattvas*. *Maya* is the limiting, Self-forgetting power of the infinite. It is the abode of finite beings and the realm of diversity.

mind A synonym for both *chitta*, the entire three-component mental apparatus, and for *manas*, the limited mind.

monism (monistic) A philosophical system in which reality is conceived of as a unified whole. (Syn., *nondualistic*.)

moksha Liberation.

mudra Seal of unity; indelible mark. From *mud*, "joy," and *ra*, "to give." Yogic postures, often hand-gestures, which are used as an aid in concentration. Also, that which gives or signals the attainment of specific spiritual states.

mukti Liberation.

n

nada The first movement of *Shiva-Shakti* toward manifestation. It is the first flutter of outward creation from the still-point, and evolves into *bindu*.

In ordinary usage, *nada* means "sound." In yoga, the unstruck sound experienced as *sushumna*. When *Shakti* fills up the whole universe with the subtle energy of *Om*, she is designated as *nada*. This is the interior, inaudible, spontaneous sound. The most subtle repetition of a *mantra* (*japa*) is *nada*, an ever-surging resonance.

Nada, anahata literally means "unstruck sound." It is the sound that is not produced by an impact that goes on vibrating spontaneously within a person. There are about ten kinds of *nada*, or *Om-sound*, referred to in books on yoga. *Spanda* is the most subtle form of this. It is the awareness that appears as sound in its extroversion, and is therefore the source of all names formed of sound.

nadi The channels through which conscious creative energy and vital breath (*prana*) circulate in the subtle body. (See *ida*, *pingala*, and *sushumna*.)

nimesha Lit., "closing of the eyelid"; involution; dissolution of the world. The inner activity of spiritual vibration (*spanda*), by which the object merges with the subject; the involution of *Shiva* in matter.

nirvikalpa A state of consciousness free of thought-constructs. Knowledge without mental ideation. *Vimarsha*, as the most subtle form of ideation, would not be excluded here. *Nirvikalpa* emerges, for example, in the pause between two breaths, sounds, ideas, or things. (See also the discussion of *unmesha*.)

Nityananda From *nitya* "constant," "always" + *ananda*, "bliss," "total well-being." Eternal bliss.

o

Om The sacred syllable that is *Brahman* itself as sound; the ultimate primeval sound. (See *nada*.)

p

para The highest; the supreme (usually seen as a prefix).

parapara Intermediate stage of *Shakti*; both supreme and non-supreme; both identical and different; unity in diversity.

paravac/paravak The supreme speech, or word. Transcendent speech. This is really a type of awareness that does not behold anything but itself. It shines only as *aham*. No "other" is present. Consists of pure awareness of the real *Self*. The unmanifest *Shakti*, or vibratory movement of the divine Logos/Mind that brings about manifestation; cosmic ideation. The Word of God.

pashyanti The finest level of speech. Speech conducted by awareness alone. Speech consisting of pure awareness at the stage of partial unity. The beholding subject (*aham*) and the beheld object (*idam*) are both evident in *pashyanti*. There is no successiveness — the order of ideas dissolves. The divine view of the universe in undifferentiated form.

pingala One of the three principle channels or subtle conduits (*nadi*) for energy flow in the subtle body. (See *ida* and *sushumna*.)

prakasha Lit., "light"; the principle of Self-revelation. An untranslatable word. Just as light makes everything visible, so because *prakasha* is there, everything else *is*. The principle by which everything else is known. Conscious light.

prana The force that animates; vital air; subtle life force; the breath of life, or energy. In the human organism, *prana* has five functions, the first of which, the outbreath, is also called *prana*. Specifically, it is the vital breath in expiration. *Prana* is not mind. It is insentient. It is not like gross physical energy. It is subtle biological energy that catches the vibrations of the mind and transmits them to the nerves and plexuses. As life-force, *prana* is the natural connecting link between consciousness and its physical manifestations. By controlling the mind one can control the *prana*, and by controlling the *prana*, one can control the mind.

pranayama Breath control.

Pratyabhijna The school of thought within Trika that is the philosophy proper. It deals rationally with the doctrines, tries to support them by a process of reasoning, and refutes the views of opponents. Its first work was composed by *Somananda*, who is seen as its founder. The texts of the *Pratyabhijna* approach now constitute perhaps the greater portion of the existing writings on Kashmir Shaivism.

r

Rudra Another name for *Shiva*.

s

sadhana Pursuit of an ideal; the practice of spiritual discipline.

samadhi Lit., "resolution"; resolving, drawing together of the mind; collecting of the mind so that its fluctuations are stilled. Deep, undifferentiated absorption. There are two types of *samadhi*: "sa-vikalpa," in which the distinction between subject and object is retained, and *nir-vikalpa*, the state in which the mind merges with the object of contemplation in such a way that the distinction among the subject, object, and means of contemplation completely disappears.

samsara Lit., "movement." Existence in the phenomenal world of contradictions and dualities. The stream of experience; the world process; transmigratory existence.

samskara The residual traces of the mind lying in the unconscious; the tensions we accumulate without being aware of them.

sannyasa Renunciation.

sannyasi Lit., one who casts away, renounces; one who has let go of worldly bonds in order to devote him- or herself to the spiritual life.

Self Self-existent, pure awareness and pure consciousness, self-luminous and, according to some schools of philosophy, also self-conscious; only one Self is manifested in all minds and bodies. Synonymous with *Atman* and thus with the Absolute.

Shakti Energy of Life Itself, divine power, identical with *Shiva*. Also used to refer to *Shiva's* consort. Dynamic pulsation; the creative cosmic power that projects, maintains, and dissolves the universe; in the individual, *Shakti* takes the form of *kundalini*. The *spanda*, or creative pulsation of *Shiva* as foundational consciousness. The phases of *Shakti* are 1) *para*, highest, transcendent, undifferentiated; 2) *parapara*, the intermediate, unity in diversity; 3) *apara*, immanent, bringing about a sense of difference.

shaktipat The descent of *Shakti*, divine grace. Transmission of the energy. In the *Tantraloka*, Abhinavagupta gives three main types: swift, moderate, and slow.

shaktopaya or **shakta yoga** *Yoga* of Self-contemplation; the ever-recurring thought or awareness of oneself being essentially *Shiva*, or pure consciousness. This is a practice in constant contemplative ideation and imagination of the real nature of the *Self*. It brings identification with the supreme consciousness, and develops the possibility for the awareness of *shambhavopaya*.

shambhavopaya or **shambhava yoga** Also *shambhava upaya* and *iccha upaya* or *icchopaya*. A strategy (*upaya*) that relates to *Shambu*, or *Shiva*. One is established in the constant awareness that the universe is nothing but *Shiva*. Direct realization of the pure and divine nature of the *Self*. The mind is rested and relaxed, not forced to stop. The *Self* is realized spontaneously and intuitively, by a mere hint that one's essential *Self* is *Shiva*, even as the mind becomes free of thought-constructs (*vikalpas*).

Shambhava is known as abhedopaya, the nondualistic means of realization. No element of mental contemplation or ideation of any type is involved in *shambhavopaya*. It comes about through the one-pointed orientation of the will and reveals the nature of the other *upayas*. The method that relates to *Shiva* or *Shambu* employs nothing else but the impulse, or power, within the heart.

Shiva The Absolute; pure consciousness, the transcendent divine principle. One of the gods of the Hindu trinity, along with *Vishnu* and *Brahma*. (See *Brahma*.) The name of the divine in general; the good. *Shiva* is the one in whom all things, subjects and objects, lie. It is also the divine who cuts asunder all limitation.

Shiva Sutras The first beginnings of what has been called "Kashmir Shaivism," to distinguish it from other forms of Shaivism known and still practiced in other parts of India, can be traced to the *Shiva Sutras*. They are a collection of sutras on *yoga* attributed to *Shiva* and revealed to *Vasugupta*. The *Shiva Sutras* laid the foundation of the *Advaita* Shaivism of Kashmir, or *Trika*.

shunya Void; the state in which no object is experienced. The void of dreamless sleep. The subtle, finite, and individual consciousness of the Self experienced in *shunya*; finite I-consciousness.

siddhi Lit., "accomplishment," "achievement." Some power, usually supernatural, attained through yogic practice.

Somananda Probably a pupil of *Vasugupta*, *Somananda* started the *Pratyabhijna* approach in the *Trika* system. One of the great sage-philosophers of Kashmir Shaivism, he flourished four generations before *Abhinavagupta* and so probably lived towards the end of the 9th century C.E. His work was carried on in greater detail by *Utpala*, *Abhinavagupta*, and *Kshemaraja*.

spanda A pulsation, or throb. Divine activity; the dynamic activity of *Shiva*; primordial creative pulsation. Apparent motion that is not a motion in Shiva, which brings about the manifestation, maintenance, and withdrawal of the universe; creative pulsation.

The stir of vibrative volition. *Spanda* is neither a physical nor a mental movement but the pulsation of consciousness that vibrates in and out simultaneously. (All such descriptions are, at best, misleading.) This pulsation of *spanda* expresses itself through *tattvas*, becoming the subjective and objective awareness of "I-ness" and "This-ness."

Outward manifestation (the universe) due to the dynamic aspect of the absolute. *Spanda* is not precisely the same as *Shakti*. It is the interior manifestation of *Shakti*. It is the aspect of the changeless that has the infinite potentiality to manifest all change.

Spandakarikas One of the foundational texts of *Trika Yoga*, dealing with consciousness as vibration. What is known as the Spanda Shastra lays down the main principles of the system in greater detail and in more amplified form than the

Shiva Sutras, without entering into extended philosophical reasoning in their support. The foremost of these texts is the *Spanda Sutras*, generally called the *Spandakarikas*. The word *karika* means "a collection of verses on grammatical, philosophical, or scientific subjects."

These *sutras* are based on the *Shiva Sutras* as a sort of running commentary. They are spoken of as gathering together the meaning of the *Shiva Sutras* mainly from the point of view of *Shakti*, and are often attributed to Kallata, the chief disciple of *Vasugupta*. It may also be that *Vasugupta* actually composed the *Karikas* and taught them to Kallata.

sushumna The middle or central pranic *nadi*, or channel, associated with the spinal column. It is in the *sushumna* that we feel the flow of the life energy. (See also *ida* and *pingala*.)

sutra Lit., "thread." Hence, it has come to mean that which holds together certain ideas like a thread; a rule; a formula.

A *sutra* is a teaching tool. It is deliberately constructed to be opaque to the noninitiate, because its inner content can only be transmitted by the *guru*. It must contain the fewest possible words, must be free from ambiguity once its inner meaning is conveyed. In this sense, it must be meaningful and comprehensive, must not contain useless words and pauses, and must be a faultless expression of the truth.

svatantra Autonomous; of absolute will.

svatantrya Freedom. Free will. Unimpeded sovereignty. It is the experience of perfect freedom; the absolute autonomy of the supreme.

Svatantrya Shakti The power of freedom. A key expression of the *Pratyabhijna* terminology. Used to refer to the highest reality when intending to imply all possible aspects and powers that can be attributed to the *Self*. The term is so often used in this school of Kashmir Shaivism that *Pratyabhijna* is often called *svatantryavada*.

swami Lit., "master of one's Self"; title given to monks and religious heads of Maths (temples).

t

Tantra / Tantras   Scriptures in general. Also, *agamic* scriptures. Sacred texts of the Shaiva and Shakta schools.

The term *tantra* means simply "extension," or "warp on a loom." Eventually it was used to refer to any book that explained certain doctrines, and it finally came to be applied to the doctrines themselves. Not every *tantra* is "tantric." The *Pancatantra*, for example, is a book of Indian fables.

Tantra with a capital *T* is used to refer to a broad system of practices. In the Hindu *Tantra*, a text is *tantric* which presents itself as revealed, without attaching itself in any way to the *Vedas*. Presented in the form of dialogues between *Shiva* and *Shakti*, such texts prescribe rituals, exercises, and other means to one's awakening. *Shakti* or *kundalini* is of central importance to all forms of Hindu *Tantra*.

These texts are based on secret teachings transmitted from *guru* to disciple. They are generally written in obscure language and their revelations are dispersed throughout a given *Tantra* or various *Tantras* in order to make them inaccessible to the person not receiving the teaching through the *guru*.

Tantraloka   The most voluminous of *Abhinavagupta's* works. It deals with Shaivism in all its aspects and is a comprehensive study of the *Trika Yoga* system.

tapas   Lit., "heat" or "fervor." From Vedic times *tapas*, in various forms, was understood to be the essential element at every level of existence, from the macrocosmic to the microcosmic. A natural power, intrinsic to the structure of reality. The cosmic creative power; the inner creative heat of the individual that is the power of the sacrifice, generated by the intensity of one's inner work and devotion.

tapasya   Lit., "that which generates heat or energy"; brooding, incubation; the concentration of energy to generate creative force. In its narrow sense, the practice of difficult or demanding spiritual disciplines.

tattva   *Tat* "that" + *tva* "-ness": thatness. Truth. The very being of a thing. The nearest English equivalent is "principle." A category of reality. In Kashmir Shaivism, there are thirty-six *tattvas*, all of which are the manifestation of *Paramashiva*.

The earlier Samkhya system had spelled out twenty-four *tattvas*; Shaivism added eleven more. Paramashiva is the basic eternal reality that encompasses all the *tattvas*. (See *Shakti*, *Maya*, the *kanchukas*.)

Trika Yoga The nondualistic Shaivism of Kashmir. System or philosophy involving various triads: 1) God (*Shiva*), the energy of the divine (*Shakti*), and the individualized self (nara); 2) the knower, knowledge, and the known; 3) the three corresponding strategies of realization (*anupaya/shambhavopaya*, *shaktopaya*, and *anavopaya*); 4) the three channels (*nadis*); 5) the three main breaths. Also, the triad of 6) the highest, nondifferentiated form of Shiva (*para*), the intermediate state of identity in difference, or unity in diversity (*parapara*), and the state of difference, or differentiation (*apara*).

The triangle is a key symbol in the Trika Yoga system. The three points of the triangle of the *chakra* at the base of the spine denote the essential concepts of this system.

turya/turiya The fourth state of animation, which is identical to Self-revelation. At the differentiated level of experience, every person's consciousness expresses itself in three different states: waking, dreaming, and deep sleep. These states are exclusive. When a person is awake, he or she has no dream or deep sleep consciousness, and so on.

However, in each individual there is a fourth state that is present as the witnessing consciousness of the other three states. The ego, limited by the body, the life force (*prana*), and the mind (*manas*), has no direct experience of *turya*, even though it is always present as the background of the other states.

turyatita Beyond all states. Pure consciousness, transcending even *turya*. The awareness of *Paramashiva*, the perfect monistic "I." In this awareness, one is conscious of "I" and "I" alone, and the entire universe appears as the *Self*. *Turyatita* should not be counted as one of the four states of animation, because all other states belong to it, emanate from it, and are absorbed back into it.

u

unmesha Lit., "opening of the eye." Unfolding. Resting in the stillpoint between thoughts, images, sounds, etc.; resting in the consciousness that is the background of these things (See *turya*). This is the definition of *unmesha* according to *shaktopaya*. According to *shambhavopaya*, *unmesha* is the emergence of the highest reality when the thought constructs spontaneously and suddenly come to a stop.

Upanishads The last group of Vedic writings, which take Vedic thought to its most sophisticated level. The *Upanishads* explore human experience to understand the identification of the *Atman* with *Brahman* as the reality underlying both individual and cosmos. These are investigations into the nature of the *Self*, and range from discussions of sacrifice to more speculative inquiry into the highest reality.

upaya Means to realization. Strategy or approach.

Utpaladeva One of the philosopher-sages of Kashmir Shaivism who lived near the end of the 9th century and into the first half of the 10th century C.E. He was pupil of *Somananda*, and wrote the first work on the *Pratyabhijna* system.

v

vairagya Intense dispassion for worldliness, not colored by desire; desirelessness; renunciation.

Vasugupta One of the great philosopher-sages of Kashmir Shaivism. He lived near the end of the 8th and into the first half of the 9th century C.E. *Vasugupta* was the teacher who for the first time expounded the Shaiva philosophy of Kashmir in a systematic form. It is said that the *Shiva Sutras* were revealed to him. His pupils recorded that he lived in retirement as a holy sage in a valley near Shrinigar.

Vedanta Lit., "end of the *Vedas*." The *Upanishads*, or a philosophy based on them. A philosophical school which contains the teachings of the *Upanishads* and investigates the nature of the relationship between the Absolute, the world, and the *Self*. The most important exponent was the great Vedanta philosopher, Shankara (788-820 C.E.), with his nondualistic *advaita* philosophy.

Veda Lit., "knowledge," or "body of knowledge." From the root *vid*, "to know." Collections of ancient hymns of the Aryan tribes that entered India in the second millenium B.C.E. In these hymns, which were part of sacrificial ritual — particularly the fire sacrifice — appear the precursors of many of the later Indian deities.

There are four *Vedas*: Rig, Yajur, Sama, and Atharva. Each is divided into four parts: hymns, rituals, reflections between teachers and students in forest retreat, and *Upanishad* (lit., "sit near"; that is, sitting near the *guru*).

Vijnanabhairava The *Vijnanabhairava* is one of the foundation texts of Kashmir Shaivism. It is among the oldest *Tantras*, or *agamas*. Its goal is the integration of the individual self to the universal *Self*, and the realization of the universe as an expression of *Shakti*. The *Vijnanabhairava* was acknowledged by *Abhinavagupta* to be an extremely important work on yoga.

vikalpa Ideation; dualizing thought; differentiation. Determinate knowledge; dichotomizing thought construct.

vimarsha Lit., "experience." The Self-consciousness of the supreme, full of the powers of knowledge and activity, which brings about the world process. The nonrelational, immediate awareness of "I." Act of awareness or Self-consciousness. *Vimarsha* indicates the essential capacity of consciousness for Self-referral. This Self-referential capacity is the *shakti*, the power of consciousness.

Consciousness is *prakasha*, and its Self-awareness is *vimarsha*. *Vimarsha* is also known as *parashakti*, *paravak*, *svatantrya*, *hridaya*, and *spanda*.

vira Hero who has conquered the senses and thoughts.

Vishnu Name for the all-pervasive supreme reality. One of the Hindu trinity, representing God as the sustainer of manifestation. The personal deity of the Vaishnavas. During times of great wickedness and trouble, *Vishnu* incarnates on the earth in order to protect human beings and gods, and re-establish righteousness. There are ten such incarnations in our present world cycle, Rama and *Krishna* being the most important. In some circles, both the Buddha and Jesus are said to be incarnations of *Vishnu*.

vyapti Omnipenetration; pervasion; fusion in the whole, in *Shiva*.

γ

yoga Union. From *yuj*, "to unite." The state of oneness with the *Self*; practices and disciplines bringing the body and mind under control in order to reach this state. The communion of the individual soul with the supreme, in which communion is union; discipline leading to this communion. The transforming of human consciousness into divine consciousness.

yogi Lit., "united." One who studies and practices *yoga*, who is absorbed in spiritual practices with the sole intent of uniting the individual with the universal consciousness.

Suggested Reading

Alper, Harvey, *Understanding Mantras* (Albany: SUNY Press, 1989).

The Bhagavad Gita, trans., Winthrop Sargeant, Foreword by Swami Samatananda (Albany: SUNY, 1984).

Bharati, Aghehananda, *The Tantric Tradition* (New York: Samuel Weiser, 1975).

Chatterjee, J.C., *Kashmir Shaivism* (Research and Publications Department, Srinigar: 1st edition, 1914; 2nd edition, 1962).

Dyczkowski, Mark, *The Doctrine of Vibration: An Analysis of the Doctrines and Practices of Kashmir Shaivism* (Albany: SUNY Press, 1987).

Easwaran, Eknath, *Dialogue with Death: The Spiritual Psychology of the Katha Upanishad* (Petaluma, California: Nilgiri Press, 1981).

Gnoli, R., *The Aesthetic Experience According to Abhinavagupta* (Benares: Chowkhamba, 1968).

Hatengdi, M.U., *Nityananda: The Divine Presence*, Foreword by Swami Chetanananda (Cambridge, Massachusetts: Rudra Press, 1984).

_____ and Swami Chetanananda, *Nitya Sutras: The Revelations of Nityananda from the Chidakash Gita* (Cambridge, Massachusetts: Rudra Press, 1985).

Hopkins, Thomas J., *The Hindu Religious Tradition* (Encino, California: Dickenson Publishing Company, Inc., 1971).

Kramrisch, Stella, *Manifestations of Shiva* (Philadelphia: Philadelphia Museum of Art, 1981).

_____, *The Presence of Shiva* (Princeton, New Jersey: Princeton University Press, 1981).

Larson, Gerald James, "The Aesthetic and the Religious in Abhinavagupta's Kashmir Shaivism," *Philosophy East and West* 26, April, 1978, pp. 236-39.

Maharthamanjari, French translation by Lilian Silburn in *Le "Maharthamanjari" de Mahesvarananda, avec des Extraits du Parimala* (Paris: E. de Boccard, 1968).

Mishra, Kamalakar, *Kashmir Shaivism: The Central Philosophy of Tantrism*, (currently in press).

Muller-Ortega, Paul E., *The Triadic Heart of Siva: Kaula Tantrism of Abhinavagupta in the Non-dual Shaivism of Kashmir* (Albany: SUNY Press, 1989).

O'Flaherty, Wendy Doniger, *Asceticism and Eroticism in the Mythology of Siva* (Delhi: Oxford University Press, 1975).

Padoux, A., "The Fourfold *Upayas* According to Abhinava's *Tantraloka*," in *Abhinavagupta and the Synthesis of Indian Culture* (currently in press).

_____, *Le Symbolisme de L'energie de la Parole dans Certains Textes Tantriques* (Paris: E. de Boccard, 1963).

Pandey, K.C., *Abhinavagupta: An Historical and Philosophical Study* (Benares: Chowkhamba Sanskrit Series, 1, 1935).

Potter, Karl, *Presuppositions of India's Philosophies* (Westport: Greenwood Press, 1976).

Pratyabhijnahrdayam: The Secret of Self-recognition, trans., with introduction and notes by Jaideva Singh (Delhi: Motilal Banarsidass, 1963).

Rastogi, Navjivan, *The Krama Tantricism of Kashmir: Historical and General Sources*, vol. I (Delhi: Motilal Banarsidass, 1979).

_____, *Introduction to the Tantraloka* (Delhi: Motilal Banarsidass, 1987).

Sanderson, Alexis, "Saivism and the Tantric Traditions," in *The World's Religions*, ed., Steward Sutherland, Leslie Houlden, Peter Clarke, Friedhelm Hardy (London: Routledge, Kegan Paul, 1988).

Sharma, L.N., *Kashmir Shaivism* (Benares: Bharatiya Vidya Prakasana, 1972).

Silburn, Lilian, *Kundalini: Energy of the Depths*, trans., Jacques Gontier (Albany: SUNY Press, 1988).

Siva Sutras: The Yoga of Supreme Identity, trans., with introduction and notes by Jaideva Singh (Delhi: Motilal Banarsidass, 1979).

Spandakarikas, trans., with introduction and notes by Jaideva Singh (Delhi: Motilal Banarsidass, 1980).

Swami Chetanananda, *The Breath of God* (Cambridge, Massachusetts: Rudra Press, 1988).

_____, *Dynamic Stillness, Part One: The Practice of Trika Yoga* (Cambridge, Massachusetts: Rudra Press, 1990).

_____, *Songs from the Center of the Well* (Cambridge, Massachusetts: Rudra Press, 1985).

Swami Rudrananda (Rudi), *Behind the Cosmic Curtain: The Further Writings of Swami Rudrananda*, ed., John Mann (Arlington, Massachusetts: Neolog Publishing, 1984).

_____, *Rudi: In His Own Words*, Swami Rudrananda (Cambridge, Massachusetts: Rudra Press, 1990).

_____, *Spiritual Cannibalism*, 3rd ed., Foreword by Swami Chetanananda (Cambridge, Massachusetts: Rudra Press, 1987).

The Thirteen Principle Upanishads, trans., Robert Ernest Hume (New Delhi: Oxford University Press, 1977).

Utpaladeva, *Shaiva Devotional Songs of Kashmir: A Translation and Study of Utpaladeva's Shivastotravali*, trans. and study by Constantina Rhodes Bailly (Albany: SUNY Press, 1987).

Vijnanabhairava or Divine Consciousness, trans. with introduction and notes by Jaideva Singh (Delhi: Motilal Banarsidass, 1979).

Index

About the Author

Swami Chetanananda is an American meditation master. He was principally trained by Swami Rudrananda, an American disciple of Bhagavan Nityananda of Ganeshpuri, a rare, gifted being of incredible yogic power and capacity. This rich fusion of East and West gives Chetanananda a distinctive voice. Even though his teaching is firmly rooted in the non-dualistic Shaiva tradition of Kashmir, his experience and his expression are thoroughly Western: Chetanananda's analogies are as likely to feature basketball's Larry Bird as the gods and goddesses of Indian myth. He has the ability to translate the often arcane and obscure elements of ancient Indian thought into a lively, familiar idiom and to apply its principles to such modern issues as lifestyle, career, and relationships.

The Nityananda Institute, headquartered in Cambridge, Massachusetts, is dedicated to the active practice of a spiritual life based on Chetanananda's teachings. A dynamic core community of over three hundred participating members take part in a daily meditation practice. Classes in meditation, chanting, and hatha yoga; studies in Trika Yoga and Kashmir Shaivism; and cultural events from classical sarod concerts with Ali Akbar Khan to lectures by renowned Sanskritist Navjivan Rastogi are offered to the public throughout the year.